ANYWAY
YOU CAN

MEDICAL DISCLAIMER

The information presented in this book is the result of years of practice experience. The information in this book is general in nature and not a substitute for an evaluation and advice by a competent medical specialist. The content provided is for educational purposes and does not take the place of the doctor-patient relationship. Every effort has been made to ensure that the content provided is accurate, helpful and understandable. However, this is not an exhaustive coverage of the subject. No liability is assumed. You are responsible for your own health.

The stories in this book are true. Grandma Rose is Dr. Bosworth's mother. The other patients' stories were told in truth with the exception of their names and circumstances to protect their anonymity.

ISBN-13: 978-0-9998542-3-5 (MeTone Life)
ISBN-10: 0-9998542-3-2
LCCN: 2018901163

For permission requests, write to the publisher, at
"Attention: Permissions Coordinator," at
hello@metonelife.com

Published in the United States by MeTone Life, LLC
3204 Madelyn Ave, Sioux Falls, SD 57106

PRAISE FOR *ANYWAY YOU CAN*

Luke Tunge – O'Gorman High School Freshman

My parents were surprised at how little instruction it took for me to catch on to ketosis. I had never been on a diet before. I got excited about the keto diet when I read the science and logic behind ketosis contained in this book. Its benefits made perfect sense to me. My parents saw how I was able to follow the diet and achieve results with foods we already had at home. As I continued this diet, my parents became interested as I told them about the mental and physical benefits and all of the diseases that can be prevented by following simple ketosis rules. I think that this simplicity in healthy eating is something that we all need, especially in the seemingly senseless, health food frenzied world.

Kerri Tunge - Mom

I read Dr. Bosworth's book after my 15-year-old son got so motivated about the keto diet after reading it. I knew it had to be more than a boring diet book if it held my son's attention. When I started the book, the story of Dr. Bosworth's dedication to her mom was so beautiful. Beyond words for me. My dad passed away from leukemia at age 65. I love that she helped her mom fight instead of letting cancer get its way.

Kim Fischer, MD - Physician of OB/GYN

Great read. I've known Dr. Bosworth for over 30 years. Leave it to her to tell a compelling true story and incorporate the complex science behind ketosis into a meaningful, easy to understand explanation.

Ryan Meyer- Business Owner

I am about as average as a person could get and reading isn't my favorite hobby. Still, right from the start, this book held my attention. I enjoyed the personal story that provides the main structure of this easy to understand the book.

I have read multiple articles on Keto and other diet topics that were nearly impossible to understand. This book certainly reaches out to a wider variety of people. This book motivated me to actually start this diet. Overall an excellent read!

Douglas Tschetter- Teacher

This is not the kind of book I would have read on my own. As a retired literature teacher and debate coach, I have spent my life reading mostly fiction and dramas and current events. As a diabetic, I probably should have read books like this, but I didn't because I lacked the interest and understanding.

I found the segments on Grandma Rose to be the most interesting. I empathize with Grandma Rose as she braved through strict food restrictions and fasting. Each segment where she sustained the restrictions amazed me. Grandma Rose actually thrived! Dr. Bosworth called her Mary Poppins, I kept thinking she's more like Wonder Woman! Those sections about Grandma Rose kept me wanting to read more because I wanted to know how she responded to the treatment she was receiving. The Lessons from Dr. Bosworth and diagrams helped me understand both the basics and inner workings of the keto diet.

Grandma Rose gives me hope.

Jennifer Rosenstiel

Before I read this book, I knew about ketosis because my husband had started it several months ago.

Dr. Bosworth's book is very easy to read thanks to the combination of facts and the personal story of Grandma Rose. It presents a realistic picture of how challenging yet rewarding the keto diet can be. Its list of starter food items and dishes is very helpful.

I did not feel like it was too technical. But if someone were looking for facts and figures they are all here. For weeks after reading the book, I continued to think about the steps I could take to improve the health of my family by what I learned in this book.

Pete Hansen, Drum Teacher & Adventurer

My family tried out Dr. Bosworth's advice in this book and here are our results:

My father-in-law, a type 2 diabetic, no longer needs any meds.

My wife and her mom got to their ideal body weight.

This book outlines and explains what the body can do when using the best fuel. Indeed, my best friend survived 4 days in the arctic racing with these book's principles. In a world with so many over-medicated suffering people, Dr. Bosworth shows you how to eat your way back to health.

Dr. Bosworth let's you in on her personal struggles as she helps her mom fight for life. This book chronicles a journey of fear, humor, determination, and science as she walked her mom through each stage of chemo treatment. Her story taught me so much about how to think about my health and living a full life.

Dawn Aspaas, Realtor

I love this book! A book that helped me understand keto basics. It made me comfortable enough to start a Keto health plan... with an inspiring story of Grandma Rose and her cancer survival story! Thanks, Doc!

Terry Kjergaard, Journalist

Dr. Bosworth knew me for years before she invited me to her keto group. She attended my retirement party. I was 370 pounds, My lungs were half-filled with water because my heart could not keep up with my massive weight. She invited me to her keto support group after a clinic appointment. She said the sugar in my veins was making my brain worse every day.

I thought I could not do it. The support group said I could. I tried. I succeeded one day at a time.

If you want to change the way you look and feel, read this book one page and carb at a time. It can change your life and save you from all sorts of health problems.

Bette Mathis, Retired Nurse

I learned how this lifestyle change can help my husband and I get healthier. It's written so that I can understand it. As we enter our 80s, this book gave me hope that we can do this. I loved her personal and real story.

Mark W. Brown, Lt Col, USAF (Ret)

I read Dr. Annette Bosworth's book hoping to find a new method to achieve weight loss through a process called Ketosis. This book helps the overweight, those with high blood pressure, ringing in the ears and numerous other health problems to include some forms of cancer. People prolonging health problems through medications owe it to themselves to read this book and learn how Ketosis can help them with a long term solution to better health. Dr. Bosworth did an excellent job of keeping the medical terminology understandable to the average reader.

Rose Bosworth, Mary Poppins

I am "Grandma Rose." This book shares my personal story. Its step by step instructions along with the daily visual ketosis testing kept me on track. Dr. Bosworth literally saved my life. Follow the rules she lays out & it will change your life too! God rewarded me with a daughter that serves the Lord in all she does. I am so blessed to be her mom.

This book is dedicated to my husband, Chad Haber. Thank you for the love and strength you give our family. Your leadership within our home makes my leadership beyond our home possible. You are proof that God loves me.

—To Those Living With Cancer, Don't Give Up—

For every book sold, one dollar will be donated to not-for-profits giving direct support to those diagnosed with cancer, including Aurora County Cancer Fund.

ANYWAY YOU CAN

DOCTOR BOSWORTH SHARES HER MOM'S CANCER JOURNEY: A BEGINNER'S GUIDE TO KETONES FOR LIFE

Annette Bosworth, M.D.
Dr. Boz®

Table Of Contents

Lessons from Dr. Bosworth:
DON'T READ THIS FIRST:
THE SECRET TO FAST WEIGHT LOSS

Grandma Rose: THE KNOCKOUT ROUND

BONUS SECTION:
7 STEPS TO STAY THE COURSE

Chapter 1

#GrandmaRose

Patients line up day after day asking me to solve complicated medical problems. We look at their problem together and we, doctor and patient, come up with a plan. After I've laid out their options, patients often ask me "Doc, what would you do? How would you deal with this?"

On a good day, I step into the patient's shoes and answer that question. It isn't easy. My training and medical textbooks programmed me with plenty of sterile 'safe' answers. Revealing what I would personally do places me out on a limb. Risking a distant fall away from the trunk and roots of conventional medicine, sometimes I bravely answer what I would personally do in their situation.

These are the moments that bring patients back to my office again and again. They thank me for showing them the path I would take.

Grandma Rose's story is a case in point.

Grandma Rose is my mom. I could fill countless pages sharing stories of how generous, forgiving, strong, and faithful she is. She shares the gift of always seeing the very best side of any human being. Come to think of it, thirty pages would not capture the depth and width of her goodness. Grandma Rose is a true-to-life Mary Poppins.

In 2007, Grandma Rose's perfectly healthy 63-year-old body failed her. Her New Year's Eve trip to the emergency room rattled our family when an infection of her lower intestine derailed her practically perfect life. ~~Mary Poppins~~ Grandma Rose left the hospital with veins pumped full of antibiotics and a thick medical chart stamped with the words: Chronic Lymphocytic Leukemia-CLL for short.

This type of lymph cell cancer lingers around the body taking refuge in places that you can't see or feel. This cancer perfectly suits the manners of Mary Poppins. No need to make a fuss with lots of symptoms and noise. Like Mary Poppins, CLL grows silently and asks no one for permission.

CLL lives in bone marrow and lymph cells. If you try to eliminate CLL with chemotherapy or radiation, these cancer cells will outsmart you. Instead, you must watch and study CLL over time, waiting for just the right opportunity to hit it at its weakest point. CLL wages an intelligent, drawn-out war, collecting battle points over time.

These battle points are tallied by way of the number of cells on each side. Good versus Evil. Healthy versus Deformed. A black and white score. The good, healthy white blood cells use their slick, flexible, nimble skills to hunt down any invading organisms that sneak into our bodies. The deformed white cells of CLLs are wrinkled, stiff, and useless. Too many CLLs and Grandma Rose dies from an infection.

The score in 2007 was Grandma Rose (GR): 1 vs. CLL: 50.

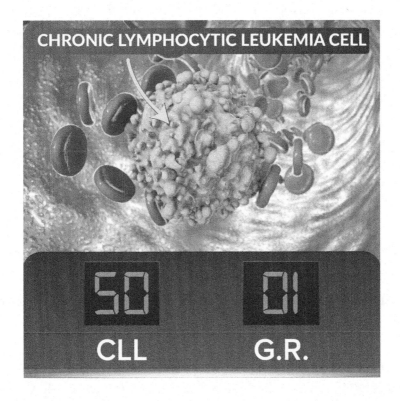

Despite those odds, her healthy white cells were powerful enough to keep her from seeing doctors for nearly 2 years. In 2009, she met her match when a mosquito bit her. That mosquito infected her with West Nile Virus. Her CLL-to-normal ratio pitted 89 deformed cells for every 1 healthy white blood cell. With those odds, she couldn't rally a defense against this invading virus.

The virus easily wove and dodged the healthy cells by hiding behind deformed ones. Within a day, the infection got to her brain: West Nile meningitis. With a swollen infected brain, she hung on to the edge of life. Two months passed before she fully recalled how to use the sewing machine that stitched all of my childhood clothes.

Over the last decade, the GR versus CLL battle points surged repeatedly to dangerous levels. Each time she got close to the edge of defeat, we beat back her CLL numbers. In those times, we reset the battlefield through chemotherapy.

Doubling rate. This term describes how long it takes for CLL to double. At first, Grandma Rose's doubling rate was two years. Then her CLL grew smarter and started doubling every six months. We thought Grandma Rose had seen the worst. Nope. It was only the beginning. Shortly after, her CLL doubled every six weeks.

We pulverized her CLL with chemotherapy. It destroyed the deformed cells and brought the CLL score down to normal. The problem with nuking her cancer cells is that we also zapped Grandma Rose. The treatment left her close to defenseless against the viruses and bacteria that naturally lived in her system.

Previously, Grandma Rose's robust immune system quickly and quietly handled any invasion. Five decades as a farmer's wife stimulated her body's defenses thanks to routine exposure to the grime of hogs, cattle and farm waste. After chemotherapy blasted her cells, she needed to stay on antibiotics for weeks to fight even the weakest of infections.

The therapy crippled her immune system. Grandma Rose teetered on the edge of collapse. Badly weakened, she slumped through the next six months just to feel half-normal again. Sapped and ashen, Grandma Rose swore she'd never do chemotherapy again.

I prayed for her to forget her traumatic chemo experience.

Three years later, we faced the same decision. Her will to fight had deteriorated. Sickly, at 67, I coaxed her into another round of chemical trauma. The army of deformed lymph cells crumbled under the power of those anti-cancer compounds. Sadly, so did Grandma Rose.

This time around, her infections broke out stronger and faster. Her lingering bacteria remembered those antibiotics and outsmarted them. We swapped antibiotics to keep the bugs guessing.

Still, after dozens of different types and kinds and combinations of antibiotics, Grandma Rose got sick. Very sick. She got so bad her CLL ratio collapsed to 1000:1. That's right-1,000 deformed lymph cells for every healthy one!

She crawled through the next six months. This time she felt half of her half-normal.

I warned my brother and sister, "I don't know how we're gonna talk her into a third round of chemo should she need it."

And there we were again in 2016. The numbers didn't lie. Her CLL count doubled every two months. She needed her chemical cocktail again. This time she was 71. Ten years of cancer smoldering within her had aged her.

It wasn't for lack of trying on her part or mine. She hung on to that resilient Mary Poppins attitude.

I reviewed every bit of information I could find about her type of cancer. I read about the new research regarding CLL. I read old literature about CLL. I sorted through both conventional and alternative therapies. I grabbed hold of every article, podcast, and editorial I could find. I wept. I prayed. I kept up with any new symptom she experienced or any change in her aging body.

Still, none of that took away the fact that Grandma Rose was now a wilted 71-year-old woman filled with cancer. She was carrying 50 extra pounds and had an immune system that matched that of a 130-year-old.

We were in trouble.

As her CLL numbers rose, the doctor ordered a repeat blood test in 8 weeks.

In April 2016, I listened to a Tim Ferriss podcast interview where he interviewed Dom D'Agostino, Ph.D. about his research on cancer and ketosis. In fact, I listened to it several times and followed my curiosity into the deep dark mysterious tunnel of this topic. The research drew me in and I couldn't think about anything else for weeks.

Convinced of the powerful potential of ketones, I put myself on a ketogenic diet on Memorial Day 2016. Truth be told, I put myself on it a month before, but I failed to produce one stinking ketone that first month. It took me four weeks to get the rules straight.

I cut out every carb I could find. I threw out all the junky carbs that were in my house because I was rotten at resisting them. During that failed month, I checked urine ketones expecting a quick victory. After a week of randomly checking and failing every time, I started checking every morning and night. Nothing. Embarrassed by my failed attempts, I parked my stubborn ego at the door and asked for help. I included my husband in removing even more high carb foods from the pantry. Together we agreed not to buy any more.

I circled back to my favorite blogs and books and it appeared I was making a very common mistake: not eating enough fat. I committed to eating even more fat. I loaded up on heavy whipping cream and butter at every turn. Coconut oil lined all of my frying pans and I even added these fats to my coffee. Finally, I produced my first ketone on May 30th, 2016-thirty days before Grandma Rose's follow up blood test.

Once I started making ketones, I worried about all that fat I ate. The rules I'd taught patients for two decades clashed with the amount of fat needed for ketosis. I resisted my habitual aversion to fat. I needed to see this chemistry experiment through. The first week of ketosis sold me.

Weathered and tired, Grandma Rose met me at the doctor's office. Her decline contrasted sharply with the surge of energy I started to enjoy when I cut down on carbs. We showed up at the appointment and her numbers announced the ugly truth: CLL 5000: GR 1.

Dr. McHale's words hit me like a slow-motion train wreck, "Rose, it's time again."

"You must undergo chemo soon or there won't be any room in your bone marrow for healthy cells. The CLL already claimed 98% of your bone's real estate. Before long, it will conquer all."

Her gaze speared across the exam room and hit me in the throat. Her eyes told me she didn't want to do this again. Tears filled my eyes as I silently pleaded with her not to give up. Selfishly, I wasn't ready to stop fighting her cancer, but this fight was not mine. No matter how much I wanted her to keep pushing, if she surrendered it meant I surrendered with her.

Twice before we had left the oncologist's office with that slip of paper. It read: "Schedule for infusions of chemotherapy."

I broke our silence with an unexpected plea. "Mom, put off chemotherapy for six weeks and let me show you what I would do. Give me six weeks."

This book shares the story-mistakes and all-of our journey to a ketogenic lifestyle. It begins with the fear of cancer but leads to so much more. My cancer-filled, 71-year-old mother's experiences fill these pages with what we learned.

When it came right down to this question, "Doc, what would you do if the person you loved the most was dying of cancer?"

My answer, "FIGHT IT **ANYWAY YOU CAN.**"

Chapter 2

Dr. Bosworth: CURIOSITY WHISPERED

Have you heard the word 'ketosis?' This weird word has been creeping into the airwaves.

I last heard this odd term back in medical school. While covering the ICU, a patient with Type 1 diabetes injected the wrong amount of insulin over and over until he slipped into a coma.

Yep, that's the last time I heard the word ketosis. Naturally, my first thoughts around ketosis link to a very sick patient. So why am I hearing this word again?

Has there been some sort of earth-shattering breakthrough? Embarrassingly, this excitement about ketosis isn't due to any new scientific discovery. This 'newfound' enthusiasm for ketosis and anything ketosis-related involves renewed media interest. Sadly, this otherwise old information still remains obscure and seems 'exotic' to nearly every doctor I know.

Brace yourself. This book represents a massive sea change in how your doctor and the whole medical community will be talking to patients about cancer, weight, health, heart disease and aging brains.

My husband is not a doctor. Twenty years of marriage to a physician specializing in internal medicine granted him a front row seat to all sorts of healthcare-related stories. He has seen the greatest benefits in the healthcare industry, as well as its ugliest traits. He has seen the flawed thinking behind doctors over using the latest and greatest procedures to cut out a problem instead of teaching patients the roots of their issues. For years, he told friends if you have an enemy that you want dead, just find out what day he is seeing his doctor. Accuse the doctor of being lazy right before your rival's appointment. Most doctors will overreach with more tests and procedures compensating for that insult. Those extra tests and procedures would be the beginning of the end for your enemy. How come? The resulting barrage of tests and procedures, paired with insufficient wisdom and patient insight, can easily become a one-way street to worse health.

The future approach I see doctors taking, mirrors the holistic approach represented in this recent revival of ketosis literature. Personally and professionally most medical practitioners haven't thought, taught or recommended ketosis. A significant percentage of medical professionals are now just waking up from the long deep hypnotic sleep Big Pharma has put us under. We're now only collectively waking up to the amazing range of health benefits low carb high fat diets bring to the table.

KETONE TERMINOLOGY

KETONES	Water soluble substrate that supplies high amount of energy to cells. Comes from fat breakdown.
KETOSIS	Metabolic state where ketones are readily available for fuel within the body. Blood levels >0.5 mmol/L
NUTRITIONAL KETOSIS	Ketosis achieved through dietary restrictions of carbohydrates. Blood ketone levels range between 0.5-3.0 mmol/L
KETOACIDOSIS	Dangerous, life-threatening metabolic state where excessive ketones are produced out of control within the body. Blood ketones soar >10.0 mmol/L causing the pH of the blood to become very acidic. Occurs in Type 1 diabetics.
KETO-ADAPTATION	State of sustained ketosis where ketones fuels the body for several weeks. The body switches to ketones as its primary fuel source. Most cells have adapted the cellular tools needed to access this fuel type.

Look at that. I already need to correct myself. That ICU patient didn't have ketosis; he had ketoacidosis

Ketosis: good.
Ketoacidosis: VERY dangerous.

Ketoacidosis is a life-threatening problem where the body's ketone levels skyrocket leading to a coma. Thanks to the quick thinking and clever technical work of our medical team we were able to avert that disaster.

Prior to seeing that patient, the only other time I had heard the term ketosis was its use as a treatment of last resort for juvenile seizure patients.

Seizures take a heavy toll on children's brains. Doctors and scientists cringe every time a youngster suffers a seizure. Each seizure kills a tremendous amount of brain cells. Some kids go through hundreds of seizures in a day. It isn't an exaggeration to say that these patients' brains are broken.

Doctors' first line of treatment involves prescribing a range of anti-seizure medications. If the seizures don't stop, we add even more meds. We know their rapidly growing brain depends upon how quickly we can stop all seizures. We try several medications in combination. When all that fails, we give up and put them on a diet that produces compounds called ketones. The goal is to get these patients to enter a state of 'nutritional ketosis.' In this state, the human body lives on fat.

In all my long years of training, my only exposure to the ketosis diet involved its use as a seizure treatment of last resort.

So what made me go back and study this again? What forced me to get curious enough to not only recommend it to my patients who've suffered from addiction, Parkinson's, Alzheimer's, strokes, and depression but adopt it for myself and my own family?

What made me curious enough to recommend it to my mother-a 71-year-old cancer patient at the time?

What made me recommend it to my sons, ages 11, 14, and 16?

What made me start this scientific and medical advocacy which completely derailed and then transformed the way my internal medicine clinic runs?

I've written this book to share these answers with you.

The seemingly overactive hype regarding ketosis turns out to have a lot going for it. In fact, there is a tremendous amount of medical literature and long-standing scientific research for why we all should be eating 70-80% fat.

If you're looking for one of the most effective and efficient weight loss solutions I've seen in my 20-year medical career, this book is for you.

If you're looking for a way to supercharge your mental stamina, this book is for you.

If you're looking for the best anti-inflammatory on the planet-100 times more potent than ibuprofen and 10 times more powerful than any steroid I prescribe, this book is for you.

If you worry about cancer and wonder why I instructed my 71-year-old-mother living with cancer to produce ketones, this book is for you.

If you would like to know why I stopped prescribing Prozac as a first-line depression treatment and started teaching patients about ketones, this book is for you.

If you want to learn about ketosis in plain English, this book is for you.

This book does not go into the complicated biochemistry and advanced science behind ketosis' benefits. I don't want to confuse you by overloading you with data. And there's plenty of it out there. Instead, I have read and re-read those sourcebooks for you and present their findings in plain language. I have worded this book in the same way I speak to my mom … the same way I teach my patients in my clinical work.

I owe a great deal to those authors and scientists who educated me through their research, lectures, and writings. There is a wonderful place on your bookshelves for their books. Instead, this book is written specifically for patients curious about ketosis and how it can work for them. It offers a practical guide to adopting a ketogenic lifestyle.

Keep reading:
- if you look down at your midsection and can pinch fat
- if you would like to know how this treatment can improve your brain, body and energy levels
- if you wish to learn how to cut down on doctor's office visits.

This book is for you.

Chapter 3

Dr. Bosworth: MD ANDERSON + D.O.D. + DEAD PEOPLE

I first became curious about ketosis in 2015.

I am a medical doctor that specializes in internal medicine. This means I focus on patients' 'long game.' I think about questions like:

What are the consequences of 20 years of high blood pressure?

What happens when you have been overweight for 15 years?

What are the risks of smoking marijuana for 10 years?

I aim to help patients prevent disasters before they ever become aware of a symptom. Thankless in many ways, but rewarding in a strategic kind of way. I specialize in helping patients achieve behavioral changes that eventually add years to their lives.

I also like to study chronic brain diseases: Parkinson's, depression, bipolar, seizures, addiction, anxiety, high blood pressure, strokes, and brain fog. My practice displays a calico pattern of patients whose brains aren't working properly.

In 2015, M.D. Anderson Got My Attention

M.D. Anderson is the world's most renowned cancer treatment center. If you are the Queen of England and you get cancer, you get the best treatment money can buy. Mayo Clinic is on your speed dial. You will receive the royal treatment for your cancer wherever you go.

However, if you have one of the 'bad boys'-I'm talking about cancers that kill people within six months-even if you get sent to Mayo Clinic they will just refer you to the crown jewel of all cancer treatment centers: M.D. Anderson. This organization leads the world in innovative ways of dealing with cancer.

When M.D. Anderson releases a cancer patient protocol, the medical world should sit up and pay attention.

Strangely, M.D. Anderson did not announce their newly implemented ketosis protocol at any medical conference. I did NOT read about this update in any medical journal.

Nope.

Instead, a patient whispered this information to me. It was as if she was worried about how I would respond.

This earth-shattering information, shared via my patient's small hushed voice, has since changed my whole approach to patient care.

Her mother was diagnosed with a glioblastoma, one of the worst forms of brain cancer. Her mother lived in Texas, near M.D. Anderson. Accordingly, she landed in the hands of one of the most innovative cancer treatment scientists today. When my patient was told that her mother couldn't receive the first dose of radiation until she'd been in ketosis for two weeks, the daughter did exactly what I would have done: she asked questions. Lots of them.

When she squeezed out all the information she could get from her mom's attending medical staff, she hit the library.

Still skeptical about whether her mother was getting the very best care, she brought her questions to me-her primary care physician. My response: a blank stare over the rim of my glasses as I processed the word 'ketosis.'

Not one of my stellar moments.

This happens a lot. Patients bring up a multi-level-marketing-hyped super weird chemical. They ask me what I think. Most of the time these chemicals are a waste of their money. Usually, those products' effects are so minor they won't hurt anyone. But that's not always the case, so I take the time to check them out.

This patient's ketosis question really kicked my brain into high gear.

For starters, when she said 'ketosis' my brain automatically heard 'ketoacidosis.' My mind raced back to that comatose ICU patient. Fifteen years had passed since I last encountered a ketoacidosis patient. Back in medical school, every time I took a test, they ask about this super scary syndrome of ketoacidosis.

My reflexive answer was to tell her "Hell no, that sounds scary!"

Except, this woman's mother was at the crown jewel of all global cancer treatment centers. Why would they be asking this woman to pee ketones before they zap her brain with cancer-killing radiation? Every single day they delayed the radiation therapy made her survival chances worse. There had to be more to this situation.

I bought myself some time and asked the patient for a week to research the question. My trusty researcher flooded my inbox with ketosis research linked to M.D. Anderson. Her research led to the articles that changed my whole practice philosophy.

I found the information referring to the new ketosis protocol at M.D. Anderson. It was rather technical, advanced biochemistry chatter. I got the essence of the message that cancer cells used blood sugar or glucose for fuel. Cancer cells don't use ketones for fuel. They don't have the cellular goods to use ketones.

For starters, ketones are fuel? Hmmpt. Interesting. Ketones apparently are not the super scary, acidic molecules known to send patients to the intensive care unit.

I'm sure we covered this in medical school. But that was so long ago it felt like new information to me. I had lost that fact many brain cells ago.

The articles went on to discuss that when we feed cancer-filled-animals only ketones, certain cancer cells starve. It sounded a little too good to be true. Still, I was not reading the latest self-published update from hucksters selling salts that change your eye color. This was straight from one of the world's leading cancer research institutions.

I scanned the report for side effects. Patients in ketosis undergoing radiation treatment run the risk of killing off too many problem cells at once. This can clog their filtration system with dead cancer cells.

What?

What a fantastic problem for terminally ill patients to have?! Let me pick THAT problem for my patients any day. We kill cancer TOO WELL? Awesome!

DEPARTMENT OF DEFENSE

My gem of a researcher didn't stop the search there. She sent me several other articles. One item from the Department of Defense caught my eye. As a doctor, this one resource stood out to me because the Department of Defense does NOT usually take money from Big Pharma.

Medical research requires funding. Someone has to foot the bill. Usually, that someone has a good reason to spend their money. Just figure out who funded the study-and you quickly know the results before even reading the report. Call me cynical, but this is how things normally work in the world of Big Pharma or direct-to-consumer industries.

Put it this way, if a multi-level-marketing company funds a study, don't be surprised if the report concludes that their product saves the world. What a coincidence, right? This is the reason why I don't get excited too easily when a new 'groundbreaking study' starts making the rounds. For me to get excited, I need something more, well, objective.

US Navy SEAL Seizure Protection Study

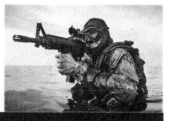

THE BENEFITS OF KETONE ESTER SUPPLEMENTS

KETONE SUPPLEMENTS :

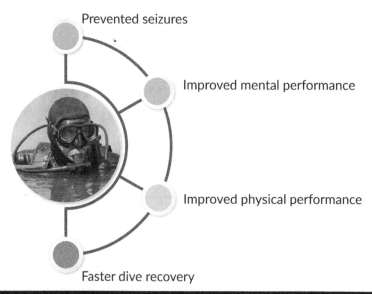

Prevented seizures

Improved mental performance

Improved physical performance

Faster dive recovery

Am J Physiol Regul Integr Comp Physiol. 2013 May 15;304(10):R829-36. doi: 10.1152/ajpregu.00506.2012. Epub 2013 Apr 3.

Therapeutic ketosis with ketone ester delays central nervous system oxygen toxicity seizures in rats.

D'Agostino DP1, Pilla R, Held HE, Landon CS, Puchowicz M, Brunengraber H, Ari C, Arnold P, Dean JB.

When it comes to objectivity, the DOD (The United States Department of Defense) does not play around. It is one of those sources where any potential bias is so small that you can almost believe every word you read.

The Department of Defense released an article describing a study involving ketosis and their divers.

At first, I thought, "How strange." Why would a deep-sea diver need ketosis? The short answer: seizures.

The resource explained that our Navy SEALS spend a lot of time under water. They also pride themselves on stealth. SEALS are all about sneak attacks. Accordingly, they don't use standard scuba equipment. Their breathing devices won't leak out bubbles. If you're trying to hide from the enemy by swimming underwater, you can't leave a trail of bubbles. Talk about a dead giveaway.

A rebreather allows divers to breathe the same air over and over again without leaking bubbles. It calculates the gas concentrations of particles in the air. Their oxygen delivery remains steady while toxic gas levels remain low.

What an awesome tool. Right? GO NAVY.

The rebreather makes stealth diving possible without a bubble trail-except for one problem: Every single one of the Navy SEALS using this device started having seizures.

Oops.

That's not gonna work. There's one thing worse than having a seizure: having one 30 feet underwater!

The DOD's research team quickly set out to discover how to prevent the seizures. The first approach they used was exactly what we used in those young kids having hundreds of seizures a day: anti-seizure medicine. They prescribed these meds to Navy SEALS. The results?

Stupid Navy Seals.

No, really.

The medicines slowed their brain processes down-by a lot. Their timing and reaction skills got super slow, and, worst of all it, didn't prevent one stinkin' seizure!

Back to the drawing board.

After reading through some literature from the 1900s, research team members found that most of the studies available focused on children. Sadly, most kids were prescribed medication that dumbed them down pretty badly. This effect, it turns out, was by design. The most common anti-seizure drugs work this way. Since seizures are spread our brain's currents, slowing down electrical activity should hold the seizures at a standstill. This solution works for most kids at quite a heavy sacrifice of mental speed and performance.

What happens when medication fails? The DOD researchers unearthed the answer: the ketogenic diet.

The fact that this report was published by the DOD made me sit up and pay attention. The results were startling. The skeptic in me wondered about the chances of this report containing your typical Big Pharma version of snake oil hype. This is, after all, the DOD we're talking about. I just could not put DOD in the same category as Big Pharma. The DOD is not exactly in the business of getting the public excited about a new treatment for seizures. There's no conflict of interest, at least, as far as I could see.

Thanks to this study, ketosis remained stuck to the roof of my mind like hard to reach mental peanut butter. Still, I was looking for something more convincing. The DOD report was eye-opening, but something still held me back from recommending ketosis to my patients.

DEAD PEOPLE

I needed another data source. Something I know that offers little wiggle room for hyped conclusions. I found it in the form of autopsies. Yes. Autopsy studies are very helpful. You set up a study selecting a set of patients who have a childhood problem and follow them all the way to death.

Once dead, look at their bodies under a microscope. That's my kind of study. Remember: I am an internist whose job is to predict what crappy things await you in the future and the best strategies to avoid them.

There is just one problem with long-range childhood to autopsy studies; They are very very very RARE. How come? This is not how most drug research is currently done. Drug companies hate these kinds of studies. They take too long and are quite expensive. To keep costs down, Pharma companies start with animal studies.

They might do a 2-year study to see how well their medicine works. From that point, a statistician makes some long-term extrapolation about future effects based on the two-year data. Blah. Blah. Blah. What's wrong with this picture? How trustworthy is data based on some goofy numbers twisted by a statistician on a drug company's payroll? Conflict-ed in their interest? Eh?

This is why the hairs on the back of my neck stood on end when my researcher drew my attention to an autopsy study involving ketosis.

Dead people don't lie ... as often.

Who are the dead people we are looking at? They were not cancer patients.

Nope, these were the kids from the 1950s and 1960s who were put on a ketogenic diet because prescription drugs failed to make their seizures go away.

Remember that one lesson I got in medical school? The one about the kids suffering from hundreds of seizures? Their seizures stopped when they started on some strange diet. Those were the ketosis kids. And now they were dying. Not from seizures mind you. They were dying of old age or health problems unrelated to seizures. When these kids were in their early teens and suffering from severe seizure disorders, their doctors had failed to control the seizures using medication.

After running out of other options, they were placed on a ketogenic diet. These kids were hospitalized and underwent ketosis transition. Even their families were trained by doctors to keep these patients on a ketogenic diet for a lifetime.

As the dead patients rolled back into the study 60 years later, a few remarkable findings appeared in the first few corpses. For starters, their brains were some of the healthiest brains the pathologist had ever seen.

Wait. Stop.

That is totally backward. These are seizure patients.

The drugs failed them. They got put on this diet as a last resort because they're having hundreds of seizures a day.

If you want to see the worst human brains, take a look at the autopsies of seizure patients who suffered decades of untreated and uncontrolled seizures. Seizure patients' brains are known for being in really bad shape at autopsy. Why are the ketosis kids' brains so different?

Even when we controlled the seizures, seizure patients' brains aged differently from normal healthy brains. They tend to be smaller. The insulation coating the nerves throughout seizure patients' brains are usually thinner. Instead of the smooth areas seen in normal brains, the brain circuits of seizure patients have a poke-a-dot pattern. Simply put, typical seizure patients' scans look a lot like some of my drug-addicted patients': broken.

These keto kids' brains were pristine.

Neurofibril tangles, also called brain plaques, are one of the disease markers we see in brains at autopsy. If you've ever looked into the grey matter of people with Alzheimer's, you'd know what a neurofibril tangle is. For those of you that haven't heard this word before, here is your crash course in neurofibrillary tangles: think of it as 'rust' in your brain. It is a buildup of 'gunk' that is linked to many brain diseases.

Brains struggling with seizures, even low-level ones, reveal many of these tangles when autopsied.

So why do the grown-up, keto kids' brains look so good?

It seems impossible. How could a seizure brain have no neurofibrillary tangles?

At this point, I became extremely curious about ketosis.

If the lack of brain damage among ketosis patients was eye-opening, my curiosity was kicked up a notch when the autopsies showed that the initial set of patients had absolutely no cancer. This was shocking to me because everybody has cancer.

Yeah, I hate to break it to you, but we all have some cancer floating around in our bodies. The real question is how well can we fight off that cancer and undo our body's cellular mistakes. If you were to autopsy an old person and tell me that they don't have cancer at all in their bodies, I won't believe you. I'd insist that you look again. I'd think that you meant that they have a lower amount of cancer. I can't imagine a human body at autopsy having totally no cancer. Everybody has a little cancer.

In the 1920s, we learned that tumor cells don't need oxygen to survive, but they certainly need glucose. Strange. Those cancer cells don't like a high level of oxygen, but they need their sugar.

Here's the clincher: cancer cells don't have the ability to use ketones for fuel.

At this point in my research, only two words came to my mind: hot diggity!!

In 20 years of practice, I've never canceled my clinic to study. Studying always came in the extra hours of running a private practice. But I found myself canceling patients so I could better understand this phenomenon I'd stumbled upon. This was far too shocking to let another day go by without my understanding, "What's the deal with ketosis?"

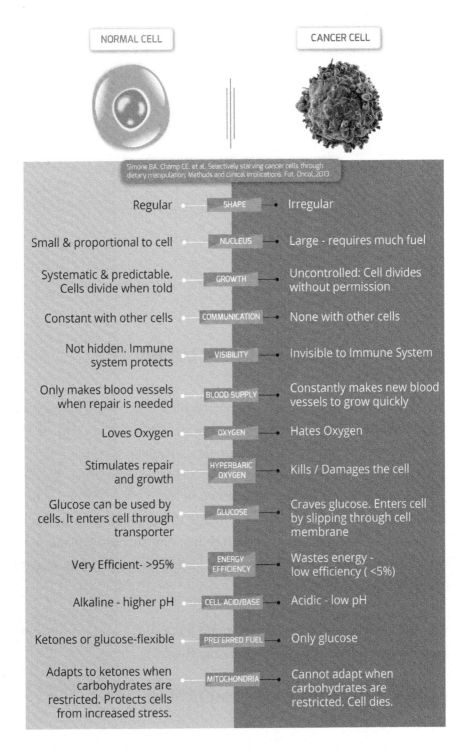

NORMAL CELL		CANCER CELL

Simone BA, Champ CE, et al. Selectively starving cancer cells through dietary manipulation; Methods and clinical implications. Fut. Oncol,2013.

Normal Cell		Cancer Cell
Regular	**SHAPE**	Irregular
Small & proportional to cell	**NUCLEUS**	Large - requires much fuel
Systematic & predictable. Cells divide when told	**GROWTH**	Uncontrolled: Cell divides without permission
Constant with other cells	**COMMUNICATION**	None with other cells
Not hidden. Immune system protects	**VISIBILITY**	Invisible to Immune System
Only makes blood vessels when repair is needed	**BLOOD SUPPLY**	Constantly makes new blood vessels to grow quickly
Loves Oxygen	**OXYGEN**	Hates Oxygen
Stimulates repair and growth	**HYPERBARIC OXYGEN**	Kills / Damages the cell
Glucose can be used by cells. It enters cell through transporter	**GLUCOSE**	Craves glucose. Enters cell by slipping through cell membrane
Very Efficient- >95%	**ENERGY EFFICIENCY**	Wastes energy - low efficiency (<5%)
Alkaline - higher pH	**CELL ACID/BASE**	Acidic - low pH
Ketones or glucose-flexible	**PREFERRED FUEL**	Only glucose
Adapts to ketones when carbohydrates are restricted. Protects cells from increased stress.	**MITOCHONDRIA**	Cannot adapt when carbohydrates are restricted. Cell dies.

Chapter 4

Grandma Rose: WEEK 1

We told the oncologist, "We need a little time. We'll be back in 6 weeks." We had this brief time until the next blood test. "Do or Die" flashed through my mind. We could do this... Right?

Despite Mary Poppins' confidence in me, I was careful not to tell anyone what we were doing. I had a fragile understanding of the ins and outs of ketosis. My failed launch before my tiny success left me with a sliver of confidence. I couldn't bear any further audience while I continued to master this subject.

We started with a garbage bag and a burning barrel. My mistakes shaped my recommendations for Grandma Rose.

START WITH REMOVING TEMPTATIONS

If you've ever helped an alcoholic throw away their hidden stash of booze, you might grasp how unsettling it was for us to dispose of all sorts of food. Grandma Rose's pantry looked like every other farmer's wife in the county: stuffed with enough processed carbohydrates to survive a famine of biblical proportions. Floor to ceiling, her shelves were filled with ketosis-killing food.

We quickly filled trash bags with cans of corn, peas, green beans, black beans, and lots of canned fruit. We tossed Bisquick, crackers, cornmeal, oatmeal, and rice. Out went wheat flour, white flour, rice flour, brown sugar, powdered sugar, white sugar, and farm-grown honey. We purged her fridge of carbohydrates hiding in ketchup, mayo, BBQ sauce, peanut butter, and low-fat milk. All the low-fat stuff like salad dressings, coffee creamers, and low-fat cheese got chucked as well. Next, we removed all baking goods like chocolate chips, evaporated milk, sweetened condensed milk, and cornstarch. Gone. All of it.

When we were done, we had three boxes of canned goods for the local charity and four trash bags full of food that no human should eat.

The pantry and storage shelves in the basement went from overflowing to barren. What was left?

Beef bouillon, pecans, and macadamia nuts. Pickles made the cut. So did green olives in oil.

We filled her shelves with coconut oil, cans of sardines, olive salad in a jar (my favorite is Muffuletta), almond butter, and liverwurst. Grandma Rose bought the biggest carton of heavy whipping cream she could find, five dozen eggs, sour cream, cream cheese, and butter. We also grabbed ketone urine strips from a pharmacy as we headed back to the farmhouse.

For ketosis to work, my parents needed to change so many habits. My folks had over seventy years of food patterns to unwind. "Do or Die."

I knew Grandma Rose would fail without a wingman for support. We recruited Dad into this high-fat-frenzy with a can of sardines. Apparently, years of mom denying him sardines was enough. "If you are telling me I can eat sardines AND liverwurst-and you say this is healthy, I am not going to argue with you."

I set their daily carbohydrate goal at 20 grams of carbs per day.

Every morning, they peed on their ketone stick and compared results. By the end of the week, both Grandma Rose and my dad crossed the ketosis threshold. Like kids, they called me to share their excitement. Seeing the positive results on their ketone strips strangely empowered them both. We were all pumped up by their initial success. So far, so good.

Chapter 5

Lessons from Dr. Bosworth:
YOUR FUEL CHOICE MATTERS

Look at what you had for your first meal today. No matter what time you first ate today, that first meal broke your overnight fast. Hence the name, 'break fast' or breakfast. Now, sort your first meal's items into these three categories:

Carbohydrates
Protein
Fat

That's it. These are the only options in life that we have. Three types of food. If you had two eggs and buttered toast for breakfast, you would have eaten all three nutrient categories:

Eggs = protein and fat.

Butter= fat.

Toast= carbohydrates.

When thinking about eating a food item, think of these three options and see which category your meal fits into. For example, if you had a bowl of oatmeal with milk, you ate mostly carbohydrates with a splash of protein. No fat in that meal.

Is it a carbohydrate?

Is it fat?

Or is it protein?

PRIMARY FUELS - Macronutrients

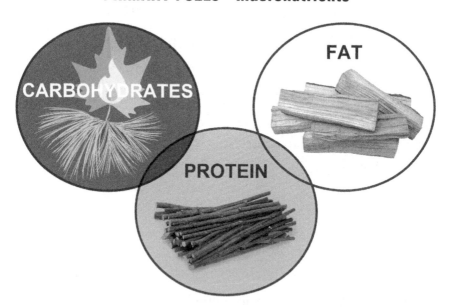

These three categories fuel our bodies. There's a whole bunch of geeky science that I can go into to try and explain this. But I'm keeping this simple. All food falls in one of these three buckets.

Let's begin with the easiest buckets: carbohydrates and fats.

Carbohydrates, also called carbs, are foods that turn into sugar inside your body. Sugar in the blood is called glucose or fructose.

Your daily energy depends on:
1) What type of fuel you put into your body
2) What chemistry was happening inside your body before you added that fuel

A campfire provides a great analogy for how different food choices result in different energy types.

Primary Fuels - Blood Glucose

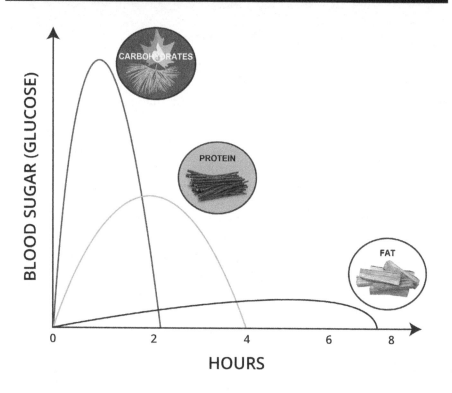

FAST & SHORT

After you rake a season of pine needles together, put them into a pile. You barely need to add a flame to watch the whole mound ignite. The dead pine needles and leaves curl from the nearby heat and burst into flames. Some even fly into the air because the process happens so quickly. And then it's over. The fuel is gone.

That's how carbohydrates fuel your body. They shoot up quickly without much trouble. The energy burns intensely but doesn't last very long. We call this a sugar rush.

What does this feel like? A sugar rush? What does a sugar rush feel like? This sounds like a silly question, right?

Yes, it may seem silly until you spend time in a clinic with patients who are unaware of their high sugar levels. These patients can drink or eat a tremendous amount of sugar without experiencing a rush.

Are you one of these patients?

You may be unaware of your chronically elevated blood sugars. A sugar rush should be easy for you to feel. Tomorrow morning, after no food or drink for 12 hours, gulp down one cup of orange juice. This should send your sugars soaring. It is like drinking a cup of sugar water. When your blood sugar peaks you should feel a surge of energy. If you are unaware of your constantly high blood sugar, you won't notice much. Your glucose levels were already high to start with, and that juice added only a tiny fraction to your total.

The price you pay for this cheap, quick fuel is the energy crash you suffer when it runs out.

SLOW & LONG

Fat also fuels your body.

Fat fuels your body the same way a brick or a solid, dense, log feeds a fire. If you've ever tried to start a campfire with a thick log as your fuel, you probably spent the night staring at a dark fire pit in the cold. Before the log would burn, it needed the correct environment in the fire pit.

The hard part about using the log is getting it started. Once you finally ignite it, you get a steady source of heat, light, and energy for the rest of the night. That's how fat works inside your body.

Fat, like the log, can be a tricky bugger to get going. But once your body starts burning fat for fuel, you get steady, sustainable, and solid energy. The heat from one burning log can spread to the next log releasing even more fuel. Fat provides a steady long-lasting source of energy for your body.

How does fat energy feel?

When you send fat into your cells' mitochondria, out come glistening compounds called ketones. Once this process begins, much like burning logs in a campfire, your fuel source becomes steady and abundant.

Drip. Drip. Drip.

MEDIUM & MODERATE

Protein energy acts like a campfire that uses twigs. The twigs produce enough of a flame to help the log or the brick churn out heat.

Without the log, the sticks quit burning. Fuel from twigs lasts longer than pine needles, but cannot sustain the fire without a log. Sticks need a steady renewal of pine needles or a continuous supply of heat from a log to keep the fire going.

If sticks burn without a log present, or without repeatedly adding kindling, the fire runs out.

If protein powers the body without fat as your primary fuel, your energy runs out. If protein molecules [sticks] are burned without fat [log] the energy [fire] runs out.

When you compare the pine needles [carbs] to the sticks [protein], the pine needles and sticks both burn pretty easily but don't last very long. The fire from the pine needles bursts much higher and faster than fire fueled by sticks but neither burns for long without help.

When you compare carb fuel to protein fuel, both delivery energy rapidly to the body, but the energy runs out. Both carb and protein fuels crash after their peak-with carbs crashing a lot sooner and harder. The sticks [protein] wear out if there isn't a log [fat] around to sustain the fire.

What does any of this have to do with a ketosis-based diet?

If your fuel comes from fat, your body makes molecules called ketones. A chain of fat goes into our cells' furnace. This cellular fuel house or furnace is called the mitochondria. It spits ketones out when fed fat. When the ketones swim throughout the body and your bloodstream, it fuels your cells with a source of energy that is steady, strong, and reliable.

Ketones show up in your system when your cells use fat, **in the absence of carbohydrates**, for energy.

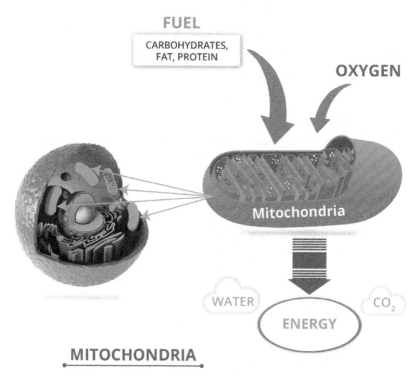

FUEL
CARBOHYDRATES, FAT, PROTEIN

OXYGEN

Mitochondria

WATER CO_2

ENERGY

MITOCHONDRIA

The "furnace" inside our cells
turns our food (fuel) into Energy

When you eat carbohydrates, glucose and other sugar molecules appear in your blood. After eating carbs, glucose, and fructose flow through your bloodstream where mitochondria suck them into their furnaces. These molecules line up in front of your mitochondria [furnace] and burn rapidly. Glucose, like pine needles in a fire, deliver fast, quick energy. Your cells' furnaces burn hot and fast when using glucose. This glucose-based energy reaches the highest heat level your body can pro-duce-only to crash when your glucose runs out.

One more time. Carbs go into your body, and mitochondria gob-ble their fast-burning, pine-needle-like energy, only to leave the system fatigued and tired after the crash. Fat goes into the body and ketones fuel mitochondria producing a steady, strong source of energy-just like camp-fire logs.

YOUR BODY'S FUEL HOUSE RULES

Rule #1: Ketosis can't begin if you have excess sugar in your blood

No fat-burning, ketone-fueled-mitochondria are activated until your sugars [pine needles] are burned through. You CANNOT use this fat-burning option if you have a bunch of sugars in your system.

Let me say that again: Glucose or carbohydrate fuel is always used before fat fuel. There is no getting around this. This rule always applies.

At first glance, you might want to call the human body lazy. Using those carbohydrates or pine needles as energy first seems like the easy way out, but there is more to the story. Our body must use those carbohydrates first. You see, too much sugar in your blood damages your body. As your sugars rise, your body will protect you from toxic sugar levels at all costs. How is sugar toxic?

Each sugar molecule attracts nearly 100 water molecules as it floats around your system. This creates a toxic inflammatory state. As your blood sugars rise and rise, so does the level of inflammation. If your system does not reduce sugars, soon every part of your body will swell with inflammation. The end results are a coma and death due to the swollen inflamed brain led by the toxic amounts of sugar.

You defend against this toxic death as you churn those sugars through your furnaces. Your blood glucose lowers along with the extra inflammation. That toxic level of sugar disappears as does the inflammation.

Rule #2: Ketosis can't begin with high insulin in your blood

When your blood sugar spikes, an alarm signal rings throughout your body warning against uncontrolled glucose levels. This chemical alarm signal is called insulin.

Insulin is the hormone your body uses to protect from toxic sugar levels and the associated swelling.

Insulin is your body's most important hormone. Nothing speaks louder and rules over more parts of the human body than insulin. When insulin circulates in the blood, sugars disappear into your cells. Insulin signals the alarm until sugar levels return to 'normal.'

How long does it take before your mitochondria switch from using carbs to burning fat for energy? Put another way, how long does it take for insulin to sink back down allowing fat to become available for your furnaces?

ANSWER: Days

Yes. It takes most American days before their extra stored sugar gets low enough for their pancreas to finally turn off its insulin faucet. High-carb diets have intoxicated your body with sugar followed by insulin. Before you can be rescued by ketone power, your sugars and insulin must drop back to normal.

Your Standard American Diet ensures that your blood pools with extra insulin. Before your mitochondria flip the switch from carb-burning to fat-burning, you have to first lower the amount of insulin in your blood. This means reduce sugar intake. Again: cut the carbohydrates.

What?   I have to go days without my carbohydrates in order to lose fat? Doc, this sounds like a starvation nightmare!!

Hang on . . . Keep reading.

Rule #3: Eat fat to burn fat

When you stop eating the carbs, your system must empty out the stored sugar you've stuffed into your liver. As the storage empties your blood sugar level creeps back up. By emptying that storage, your blood sugar stays up and that keeps triggering insulin.

It can take a couple of days before your liver storage bin is empty. No matter if those sugars come from the carbs you're eating or from storage, insulin enters the equation and always stops ketosis. The enemy of ketones is insulin. When insulin is whipping those carbohydrates around, not one stinkin' ketone circulates in your system. Insulin blocks that process until the sugars are low enough. No ketones allowed until *both* your carbs and insulin have settled down.

To exit this whole messy cycle of insulin and sugars, eat fat without consuming carbs. The one food you can eat that signals NO insulin is fat. Stop the carbs, and eat fat.

You stop releasing insulin once your sugar level drops low enough. After both your insulin and sugars are lowered your mitochondria flip their furnaces from burning carbs to burning fat. That's when you will find a trickle of ketones circulating in your system. Ketones give you steady and stable energy.

Rule #4: Measure Ketones

How will you know when your furnaces switched fuels?   MEA-
SURE IT!!

This is my favorite part.   Don't guess which fuel you're using-
MEASURE IT.   When your body is making ketones by fueling from fat,
the urine and blood will show it.   Prick your finger to check for ketones
in your blood, or more simply pee on a urine ketone stick. You can pick
these up at your local pharmacy. These sticks will quickly let you know if
you've achieved ketosis.

Let's recap.

Mitochondria produce energy throughout the human body. These
little furnaces within your cells pump out the energy your body needs.
You can choose which energy your body runs on by your choice of food.
You can choose your energy source by what fuel you put in your furnaces.

If you eat carbs, you will flood your bloodstream with glucose.
Insulin chases those sugars out of circulation and into your cells. Your
mitochondria rapidly process those carbs to produce hot, fast energy.
Much like the fire from dried pine needles, this sugar energy shoots up
and crashes down within a short timeframe. That super hot fire feels like
a rush at first, but over time that repeating flame does more damage than
good.

Stop eating carbohydrates and fuel your body with fat. Within
days, you will shift away from carb-chemistry and start burning fat.
Switching the body to ketone production will not begin until you significantly lower your sugar and insulin. While your system empties the
stored sugar from years of carb-fueling, eat fat so as not to produce any
extra insulin.

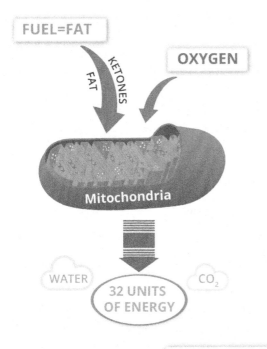

FUEL=FAT

FAT KETONES

OXYGEN

Mitochondria

WATER

CO_2

32 UNITS OF ENERGY

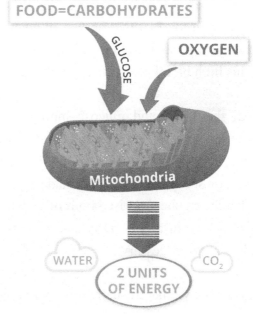

FOOD=CARBOHYDRATES

GLUCOSE

OXYGEN

Mitochondria

WATER

CO_2

2 UNITS OF ENERGY

Chapter 6
Grandma Rose: WEEK 2-6

My screw-ups from the prior month fast-tracked Grandma Rose and Dad's ketone production. With two 70-year-olds cutting all their carbs, I expected to hear complaints about the keto flu. Dad kept quiet. He was relishing the fact that he was allowed sardines and a salt shaker again. Along with his other doctors, for years I had warned him that salt worsens his high blood pressure. Keto chemistry is different.

All the sugar and glucose hiding in their 'healthy' fruits and homemade sauces stopped. At first, Grandma Rose felt grumpy and really tired. She remarked that it was a good thing the closest carbohydrate was miles away or she would not have made it through those first few days. Shortly thereafter, she surprised both of us when her energy shot up. Her habit of a cat nap in the morning and a 'dog-gone' nap in the afternoon were suddenly not necessary.

"I laid down like I usually do, but I could not fall asleep."

Dad's results were spectacular. We stopped two of his blood pressure medications after two weeks of ketosis.

My leading month of ketosis encouraged them to see the sustainability in these benefits. These changes were not a flash in the pan as long as they stayed in ketosis. I had never felt better! I could focus better at work and study for hours in the evening. This was something I thought I would never experience again.

Over the next five weeks, Dad lost nearly ten pounds. Wow!

Grandma Rose and I ate too much cream and had far too much butter to lose any weight. Surprisingly, we did not gain weight either. We put butter in our coffee. We cooked with butter. We ate vegetables soaked in butter using it as the delivering vehicle to get those fats into our guts. And it worked. We felt great. Our ketone levels were solid, never wavering out of ketosis. Every day for forty-five days we produced ketones.

FAVORITE TREAT: Grandma Rose and I had a history of ice cream in the evenings. We both knew this habit was going to be our weakness. This little recipe got us through our tempting habit. In the beginning, we used this every night just to make sure we did not fall off the keto wagon.

2 packets of Truvia
4 cubes of frozen avocados.
¼-½ cup heavy whipping cream
¼-½ cup coconut cream.
> TIP: Buy canned coconut milk. Store one can in the refrigerator. This hardens the fat-filled coconut cream part of the product and allows you to pour off the co-

conut water. Use only the high-fat portion of coconut milk.

2 teaspoons of Cacao Powder.

Cinnamon to taste

Put all of the above in a blender and puree away for the best carb-free ice cream EVER!!

Chapter 7

Lessons from Dr. Bosworth:

BAH! HUMBUG!

Why were we so afraid to tell the doctor exactly what we were doing? At first glance, you might see it as a cowardly thing to do. After all, I am a doctor that gives advice to hundreds of people. What motivated me to not tell Grandma Rose's doctor?

In a word: Time. I just didn't have any time to debate ketosis with them. Refuting ketosis objections takes time. I cover the most common of these throughout this book one "bah humbug" at a time. Some or all of these might be running through your mind as you read this. Scan through these objections and flip to the page where I answer these questions.

Objection #1: "Isn't Ketosis similar to or the same as Ketoacidosis?"

Objection #2: "The human body must have carbohydrates. We can't live without them!"

Objection #3: "Low carb causes depression. My friend did it and totally got depressed."

Objection #4: "Doc, calories matter. Why aren't you telling us to count calories?"

Objection #5: "Isn't this the diet where your body gets so whacked out that you start producing fingernail polish remover?"

Objection # 6: "Doc, I can't do keto, I have bad kidneys!"

Objection #7: "Low carb diets cause high cholesterol."

Objection #8: "What about exercise? I am training for a marathon, and use carbs, carbs, carbs for my fuel."

Objection #9: "Wait. Why was she eating 30 carbs per day? Doesn't this violate the 20-gram rule?"

Objection #10: "If I fast I will break down and start eating my own muscles."

Objection #11: "Won't this high fat diet clog my arteries and give me a heart attack?"

Objection #12: "If you eat all that fat, you'll certainly gain weight."

Let's tackle the first 2 objections in this chapter.

OBJECTION #1: "Isn't Ketosis similar to or the same as Ketoacidosis?"

Truth be told, I only hear this objection from healthcare professionals. Like me, their brain jumps to the near-death scenario of ketoacidosis. Most of my patients have never heard of either of these words. Before you present this idea to your doctor, copy this page and take it along on your visit.

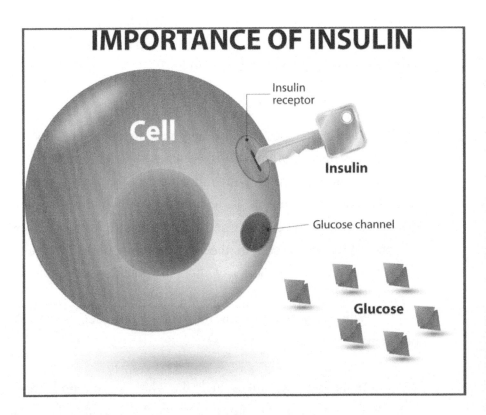

Ketoacidosis: DANGEROUS

This is a life-threatening condition. It sometimes happens to Type 1 diabetics-people who cannot produce any insulin. Their pancreas does not produce this sugar-handling hormone when their blood sugars rise. Without the injection of insulin, Type 1 diabetics can't use blood sugar as fuel. Insulin triggers your body's cells to capture the free-floating sugar in the blood and deliver it to your furnaces. Only then can your cells burn it as fuel. Without insulin, sugars circulate continually and never enter cells. Insulin is the chemical key that allows glucose to enter cells. Once inside, mitochondria burn this sugar compound for energy.

When mitochondria can't access sugar fuel from your bloodstream, your body switches over to ketones. As previously stated, the enemy of ketones is insulin. When there is no insulin in your body, ketone production has no limit.

Ketones, as fuel, work just dandy for Type 1 diabetics. Unlike glucose, ketones need no help getting from your blood to the furnaces insides of your cells. Ketones slip right through your cell walls and straight to your mitochondria for energy production. Ketones ARE usable to a diabetic. Without insulin shots, Type I diabetics switch each and every cell to a ketone-burning furnace. With every cell in the body burning logs for fuel, a tremendous amount of energy swelters the system.

With every cell glowing hot with ketone fuel, what is the problem?

As the Type 1 diabetic fuels the whole system on ketones, their body's chemistry becomes overheated and acidic. They can die from this situation. Heavy ketone buildup creates an acidic environment: keto<u>ACID</u>osis.

Ketoacidosis: DANGEROUS

For those of us that normally produce insulin, even after months of cranking out ketones, we will never have 100% of our furnaces burning ketones. Many of our cells use ketones for fuel, but some cells still use glucose. Glucose always outranks fats for fuel, as long as there is insulin present to assist the glucose with entrance into the cell. If glucose floats by, insulin triggers the cell to grab glucose and pull it in. That cell burns glucose while ketone fuel is halted. This leaves a constantly changing percentage of cells that use ketones and glucose at the same time.

Ketosis: NOT DANGEROUS

Nutritional ketosis refers to the steady production of ketones which are then converted by your mitochondria into energy. Ketosis is triggered by a sharp drop in blood sugar inside the cell. This low glucose is made possible by fasting or cutting out your carbs. Without insulin, Type 1 diabetics have low blood glucose inside the cells because they have no insulin 'keys' that allow entrance.

Here's how it normally plays out: once you stop eating so many carbs, your body uses up its stored sugar.

For those of us with insulin, our body burns the glucose fuel circulating in your blood. Next, it empties your stored fuel in your liver. When all that's used up, your insulin and sugars drop continuously. Finally, insulin all but disappears.

One by one, your mitochondria switch from glucose to ketones for fuel. They keep the fire burning, but transition from the fast-burning sugars to slow-burning fat. Not every mitochondrion makes the switch, but more and more of them transition to burning fat. A few sugars enter your system and quickly get burned as the mitochondria switch back and forth.

When you eat mostly fats, your mitochondria become efficient at using either option for energy. A few are switching over to sugar and back again to fat when all the sugar is gone. This fat/sugar blend keeps ketone levels within a safe range. Without insulin, close to 100% of your cells burn ketones. This creates the life-threatening situation of Keto<u>ACID</u>osis.

OBJECTION #2: "The human body must have carbohydrates. We can't live without them!"

Not true.

A few essential nutrients are needed to sustain life. Let's review these.

Essential For You to Live

1. WATER
2. ENERGY (your fuel)
3. MINERALS/ELEMENTS:
   MAJOR ELEMENTS include calcium, phosphorus, potassium, sulfur, sodium, chlorine, and magnesium.
   TRACE ELEMENTS: Trace elements are a little harder to find. These include iron, iodine, copper, zinc, manganese, cobalt, chromium, selenium, molybdenum, fluorine, tin, silicon, and vanadium.
4. AMINO ACIDS:
   Isoleucine, leucine, lysine, methionine, phenylalanine, threonine, tryptophan, tyrosine, valine
5. FATTY ACIDS:
   Linoleic, linolenic
6. VITAMINS:
   WATER SOLUBLE: Thiamine (B1), riboflavin B2), pyridoxine (B6), cobalamine (B12), niacin, pantothenic acid, folic acid, biotin, lipoic acid, Vitamin C
   FAT SOLUBLE: Vitamins A, D, E, K
7. MISCELLANEOUS:
   Inositol, choline, carnitine

Harper AE. Defining the essentiality of nutrients. In Shils ME et al, eds. Modern Nutrition In Health and Disease. Baltimore, William & Wilkins 1999, pp. 3-10

BIOLOGY CLASS 101:

Mammals need to consume the following things to stay alive.

1. WATER

2. ENERGY FOR FUEL

Energy can come from carbohydrates, protein, or fat.

3. MINERALS/ELEMENTS

These minerals are found throughout nature. Some of them are major parts of your diet, others are known as trace minerals. Skip out on these minerals for too long and your body will 'fail to thrive.' This is the language doctors use when we are trying to politely say, "You are dying."

MAJOR ELEMENTS: include calcium, phosphorus, potassium, sulfur, sodium, chlorine, and magnesium.

TRACE ELEMENTS: Trace elements are a little harder to find, but without them, you can't go on for long.

You only need a few bites of nutrient-dense food every week to get your body's quota of these trace elements. Once you meet these nutrients' minimum requirements, your body thrives.

4. AMINO ACIDS

Amino acids come mostly from protein and are very important for survival. Your body needs these to create and repair your tissues.

5. FATTY ACIDS

Fatty acids are fat. These come in three natural types and an extra man-made one: saturated, monounsaturated, polyunsaturated, and trans fats. The first three are all found in nature. Trans fats are not found in nature. They are produced by chemical processes to enable them to remain solid at room temperature. Your body makes most of the fats it needs from the food you eat or the energy stored inside your cells. However, two fatty acids are the exception. These two are essential for you to eat because you cannot make them yourself. These essential fats are called omega-3 and omega-6 fatty acids. Omega-3 fatty acid (a very short acid also called linoleic) and omega-6 fatty acid (a slightly longer compound called linolenic) are required for life.

Without omega-6, your body can't make the hormones that activate your immune system. Omega-3 assists in cell communication, blood clotting, contraction and relaxation of artery walls, and inflammation. Omega-3 fats are also needed for the formation of cell membranes.

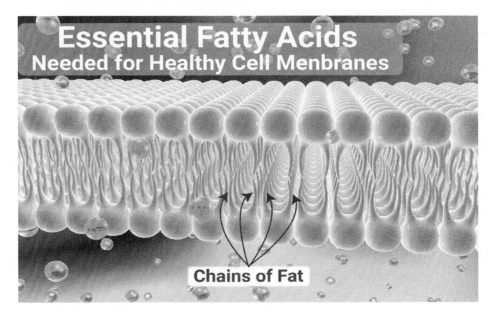

Essential Fatty Acids
Needed for Healthy Cell Menbranes

Chains of Fat

This picture shows an image of a cross-section through the membrane holding your cells together. Look closely to see the repeating structure of a sphere with 2 tails lining up in perfect formation. The tails projecting from the spheres are chains of fat. This pattern is perfect, free from defects, because of the ample supply of these 2 essential fats. If your body makes cells without enough Omega-3 fats it won't be long before you find defective and eventually cancerous cells.

6. VITAMINS

These nutrients either dissolve in water (water-soluble vitamins) or oil, (fat-soluble vitamins.) Without these compounds, your system will soon fail to function, repair and protect you.

7. MISCELLANEOUS

The 3 components left (inositol, choline, and carnitine) are also required for life. They don't fit into any of the above sections.

Did you notice something?

That's right-nowhere in the seven listed items above will you find 'essential' carbohydrates.

Nope.

None. There simply is no nutrient that we can't get from other sources if we stop eating carbs.

If you start your day with eggs, tomato, and butter, you've already loaded up on vitamins A, B, C, D, E, and K, and all kinds of other nutrients. When your mom calls and says you need to eat fruit or you will die, show her this chart. Ask her EXACTLY which essential nutrient is needed to sustain life.

You will win this argument every time.

Chapter 8

Lessons from Dr. Bosworth:
KETONES FOR LIFE

Have you ever met a toothless dentist? Have you met a veterinarian who's never owned a pet? How about a preacher who always seems worried?

It's the same problem when you meet an unhealthy doctor and her family. They're overweight, stressed, on high blood pressure meds, wearing a CPAP machine… they're just unhealthy. I can draw a sharp line sorting the colleagues who figured this out and those who haven't. The same process goes for patients. I can draw a line down my patients who have adapted to a high-fat life versus those still loading up on carbs.

KETONES FOR LIFE

When I began this adventure into the keto lifestyle, I thought almost exclusively about my mother and her battle with cancer. It was not long into my education that I lost track of all the additional benefits this high fat low carb lifestyle would have for patients. My list continues to grow. Central to all these benefits is ketosis' impact on INFLAMMA-TION.

Instead of listing the thousands of benefits ketosis delivers, I have only included the ones that surprised me. These symptoms, in large part, were taught to me by my patients.

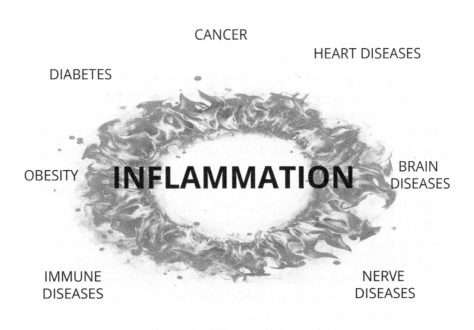

CANCER

HEART DISEASES

DIABETES

OBESITY **INFLAMMATION** BRAIN DISEASES

IMMUNE DISEASES

NERVE DISEASES

MUSCLE DISEASES

WEIGHT LOSS

The bulk of this book focuses on how ketosis promotes weight loss. From the chemistry-shift needed for those overweight to the improved energy burning inside your cellular furnaces, this diet wins for sustainable, healthy weight loss. Having said that, I still included it in this section because it surprises my patients and me how easy the weight loss is once you get ketosis figured out.

MENTAL EFFECTS

I'll be honest. This is what kept me keto. It wasn't the weight loss. Certainly, I started ketosis because of my mother's cancer, but its anti-cancer benefits aren't the reasons I kept going.

My mental sharpness keeps me loyal to producing ketones. In fact, I would have never been able to write this book if it weren't for the effects of ketones on my brain.

It's hard to believe switching to a keto diet is going to improve your mental processes-especially during the initial transition from carbs to fat. As your brain adapts to using ketones for fuel instead of glucose, you get a woozy feeling. Often, this comes with a noticeable slump in your mental processing. Your mood and mental performance dips. This can be rough. I have lost several patients to this slump when I failed to properly warn them that this gets better. As those first days lead you into your second week of ketone production, things change dramatically.

When I first became a doctor, it was very hard for me to guess how medications I prescribed would affect patients. For example, when I would write out a prescription for an antidepressant, patients would ask how long before they feel better. The right answer was, "I don't know." Different people respond to medication differently. The depths of one person's depression looks quite similar on the outside, but is indeed very different on the inside as compared to another. Some get better in two months while others take much longer. At first, I over promised the way patients would feel. I told them they would notice improvement without properly understanding how poorly their brain was working and how little the medication would do. Years of experience have taught me to carefully answer that question based on many factors unique to each patient.

When I first transitioned into producing ketones, I did not expect it would improve my mental functions or emotional well-being. I didn't suffer from depression or anxiety. I slept well. I, essentially, felt *normal.* Indeed, any claim I had heard regarding ketosis and mental improvement reminded me of those over promised expectations I spouted to patients two decades ago. By the end of the second week, I wrestled with giving credit for my improved energy, focus, and mood to the ketones coursing through my veins. Since then, I have continued to see nothing but improvement in my brain function. I feel like I am 25 years old again. I can concentrate on complex tasks for hours straight.

Walt is a 67-year-old patient of mine who suffers from alcoholism. He has struggled to stay sober for the last thirty years. The most powerful improvement Walt has ever felt came when he chose to join my keto support group. Walt's experiences with sobriety AND keto-adaptation compel me to share his testimony with all of my addiction patients.

Here is his story:

Age: 67   Height: 72 in   Weight: 270   BMI: 36.07
Blood Pressure: 4 medications to keep it in the 130s/80-90s
A1C (Average Blood Sugar): 5.8 Average Glucose= 120
HsCRP: 4.2 (normal is less than 1.0)
Reason for going KETO: Stop Drinking.

Walt is a 67-year-old medical doctor respected by his colleagues for his extensive service and skills. Walt is wicked smart and has reached the top of his profession. Six feet tall and weighing 270 pounds, his size alone commands attention. Add to this his IQ and authoritative personality and it's easy to see why many consider him a force of nature.

For 30 years, Walt's kryptonite was booze. Multiple treatment programs didn't cure him. His intelligence was hijacked by his drinking habit. He'd once celebrated three years without a drop and called it sobriety.

Unfortunately, a closer look at this 'dry' period reveals another addiction. When the alcohol stopped, the sugar started. The sugar helped him stay away from booze, but a total relapse of alcohol addiction consumed him the past three years.

The empire that he had built—the clinic with his name on it—kicked him out. Forty years ago, he founded that clinic and built the army serving the community under his leadership and name. Now, the partners voted and he was gone.

Here he was, in my clinic, 67 years old, kicked out of his career, a wife ready to walk out the door, and his health in the toilet.

Sobering up was something he knew how to do well. He had done it hundreds of times. This time, he chose not to spend another $40,000 on an inpatient alcohol treatment. He had done that many times before without success. His swollen, booze-soaked brain short-circuited with cravings. These haunted his dreams. The drinking nightmares lingered for weeks while he would white-knuckle the decision not to drink. Then one day, the part of his brain that craved desperately for alcohol would spread the message to cover every wire in his mind.

This time I invited him into our weekly keto support group. He scoffed at the idea that changing his diet would have any impact on his alcoholism. Instead of arguing, I asked him to look in the mirror. "Walt, look at you. You're 100 pounds overweight, on four blood pressure meds, you're a diabetic in denial with rosy cheeks announcing your addiction to everyone. Don't argue with me, just do what I tell you to do. If you don't feel better in four weeks under my instruction, you can have your old life back."

He surrendered. In those four weeks, he gave me 100% of his trust. By the end of his first week of peeing ketones, Walt got off two of his four blood pressure medicines. By the end of the second week, his sleeping pattern had settled into the kind of deep, restorative rest that repairs brains. Each week, his weight and blood pressure decreased. More importantly, he continued to improve mentally at a rate that I have never seen in my medical career.

In four weeks, this amazing, intelligent, driven man who wanted to commit suicide nearly every day of the prior month, had transformed. He walked into the group with a smile. Not the kind of 'public' smile that hid his sadness. He authentically felt good. Each week, his sugar and alcohol cravings lessened. His first week of sobriety was coupled with a 10-pound weight loss. Over the course of the next three weeks, he lost another 20 pounds. Most importantly, he wasn't craving alcohol.

After six weeks of peeing ketones, Walt shared this, "Doc, I know you've told me countless times that my brain will heal if I just stop drinking. It was something I heard, but never really believed. This past month has been the best my mind has worked in over a decade."

Nine months into Walt's sobriety, he told the group he felt authentically dry. He reported something had changed in a way he did not think possible. Walt lost over 40 pounds in nine months, and reversed the age of his brain by nearly 40 years. Walt plans to pee ketones until he dies.

I have walked hundreds of patients through the addiction recovery process—not just alcohol but also heroin, cocaine, nicotine, and, now, carbohydrates.

Chemically, carbohydrate addiction involves the same repeating mess we see with other addictions. You get a burst of dopamine when you eat or drink a bunch of carbohydrates. This chemical surge rewards your behavior. The resulting dopamine burst feels good. It feels so good, you start craving it. You then ingest more and more sugar chasing that dopamine high. Before long your brain is addicted. You depend upon that 'hit' of sugar to just feel normal. Without sugar, you experience a dopamine 'withdrawal' state-you feel crabby, irritable, and even depressed.

Carbohydrate or sugar addiction is as real as cocaine addiction. My patients coming off of heroin, marijuana, or alcohol experience sadness after they quit. Even if they really want to stop, they can't help but miss the object of their addiction.

The same thing happens if you eat carbs to feel better. You used carbohydrates to increase your dopamine, creating that feel-good release. You must learn a new way to achieve this feeling. Your well-being depends upon the continued production of dopamine. Food cravings melt away when you switch to a ketone-based fuel. However, this doesn't address grumpiness left over from the lack of dopamine. This remaining moodiness sabotages many people switching to a keto lifestyle. Prepare for this.

For the same reasons I recommend a peer-based support group to my alcoholics, I recommend that my patients join a support group of ketone producers. Get over the switch and claim a fuller, happier life of freedom. It's a tough transition, but it is doable.

Ketosis Also Reverses Depression Symptoms

Patients report their dreams became more vivid after successful keto-adaptation. Personally, I think many of these patients had a form of depression. Even if they resisted that depression 'label'-and I don't blame them for pushing back against the term-the improvement in their cognitive state mirrors that of recovering depression patients. Watching a patient come out of the depths of depression teaches the observer how far the brain can sink and yet quickly recover and self-repair. If I could bottle the secret formula for that awakening, I would use it hundreds of times a month in the patients I see.

My severely, chronically depressed patients waddle in the sludge of darkness and brain fog for months-even years. They struggle to make decisions. When I insist they switch their diet, even their dog groans with disbelief. A successful behavior change appears too heavy of a burden. This leads me to their caregiver. Their spouse, or parent, or even their child must lead the way to this new way of eating. Just like when I lead the way for Grandma Rose, the diet will be just as helpful for the companion as it will be for the patient.

Whatever reason they started eating 80% fat, I don't care. I am awestruck at how fast their brains become re-energized.

INSULATE YOUR NERVES BY MAKING THEM FATTER

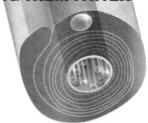

ONE LAYER OF FAT AROUND THE NERVE
Messages traveling down this nerve lose speed and focus because the insulation is too thin.

MANY LAYERS OF FAT SURROUND THE NERVE. The insulation is thicker keeping the messages traveling down the nerve properly focused and fast.

Prozac or no Prozac, I switch all of my depression patients to a ketosis diet. The results have been nothing short of impressive.

LIBIDO

WARNING: this diet will raise or normalize your hormone levels. One tell-tale sign of a hormonal surge in women is menstruation. If you are a woman of childbearing age, get ready for unexpected menstruation when you eat mostly fat.

When women switch to a keto diet, their fatty foods deliver a cocktail of rich nutrients. These nutrients, in turn, help restore depressed or problematic hormone levels. Women with normal estrogen levels report a surge in this hormone within the first week of going keto. After 3-4 weeks, my keto-adapted female patients report a significant increase in their libido.

How come?

Patient after patient brings this up. The human body's fat cells are closely linked to the production of estrogen and testosterone. Fat, specifically cholesterol, is the starting compound for many steroid hormones such as estrogen, testosterone, progesterone, cortisol, and aldosterone. Ketosis results in the conversion of a lot of body fat to energy. This process boosts hormone production as well.

I believe the increase in sex drive also happens for a different reason: ketosis' improvement of overall brain function. Orgasms happen in your brain. When your brain does not get proper nourishment and rest, your mental function starts to deteriorate. Sleep deprivation and malnourishment chronically swell your brain. A swollen brain is a broken brain. Mental processing suffers greatly with the slightest of inflammation affecting your gray matter. Libido and sex drive are related to brain function. While hormones do play a large role, your sex drive can be depressed if your brain isn't working right.

SLEEP

My keto-adapted patents report improved sleep duration and quality. Your brain needs good nourishment to function properly. Brains are made of 70-80% fat. Every circuit winding through your brain is coated with a layer of fat. On a high carb, high sugar diet, the quality of the fat your body produces suffers. The fat produced inside your brain acts as an insulation lining for each of the nerves in your brain. During periods of deep sleep, you continually repair and replenish the fat insulating each pathway.

High amounts of glucose found in the blood and brain attract water. Water and "electricity" don't mix. This water produces swelling and inflammation that disrupts brain processing. Your brain function and efficiency reduce thanks to this swelling. If there's one fatty tissue in your body you want well-nourished, it's your brain.

The quality of the fat produced daily inside your brain depends on how well-nourished your brain's fat-making cells are. If these cells are swollen and inflamed, the fat they produce is flimsy and breaks down easily. During ketosis, the quality of the fat lining your mental circuits improves, as does the depth and quality of your sleep. A swollen brain is easily fatigued, yet does not sleep well. The longer your brain is exposed to higher ketones and lower blood sugars, the better you sleep.

SKIN

Touch your face. Those skin cells you are touching were made 2-3 months ago. If you want healthy, glowing skin that's free from pimples and wrinkles, improve the quality of the skin cells you make today. Improve those cells at the base of your skin layer and watch your age reverse over the next 2-3 months.

A predictable change in your skin unfolds after 2 months of ketosis. It all begins with removing inflammation. First, your pimples fade. No matter your age, ketosis prevents pimples from popping out of your skin. Next, the skin redness, inflammation, and irritation slowly fade. Your skin will begin to glow about 90 days after you produce your first ketone. Your skin will show a youthful radiance that easily outshines the look you get from a fresh layer of lotion. Instead, this degree of youthfulness comes from a much more sustainable process. Skin cells formed during ketosis were made in the absence of inflammation. At the root of any acne problem lives a soupy mess of cells soaking in the grime of inflammation. Stop the inflammation and youthful, radiant skin surfaces several weeks later.

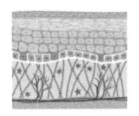 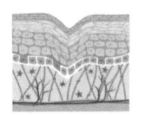 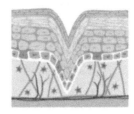

35 YEARS　　　　　　　45 YEARS　　　　　　　55 YEARS

Do you remember that part about essential fats mentioned under Objection #2? I mentioned how every cell is lined with these special fats that are essential to life. Without enough of that fat, your cell membranes fail to form the perfect pattern. There are defects in your cell membranes.

Skin cells that break, split open, or wrinkle were made with these defects in the cells. Inflammation is at the root of these problems as well. A sunburn is an example of severely inflamed skin and it's easy to see. Lower amounts of skin inflammation are not as obvious. Low-grade inflammation occurs on a microscopic level. Inflamed skin cells produce imperfect outer layers. These imperfect cells don't stack together as neatly, forming defects in the skin. These are wrinkles.

In contrast, well-made skin cells are flexible and plump allowing the cell membrane to stretch and squish as needed. As we age, our defective skin cells increase in number. These replicate and divide into even more defective cells. Defective cells tend to make defective copies. Those wrinkles around your eyes showed up in your thirties. Maybe the inflammation started after a sunburn. Maybe it built up during times of high stress. Either way, those cells wrinkled because they were defective. Ten years later, those wrinkles are deeper and more noticeable.

Would you like to make some of these flexible, radiant, youthful skin cells? Get to the root of your wrinkles, crows feet, smile lines, thinning skin and other problems of your skin. Pee ketones for 90 days.

ARTHRITIS

When burning fat for fuel, your body bathes in ketones. Your joints soak up this slick, lubricating substance reducing inflammation and friction. Ketones sneak into the tiniest spaces in your body. Our joints go through quite a bit of wear and tear. While they do have the ability to self-repair, they can only do so if they are not inflamed. I've had arthritis patients on ibuprofen for the better part of a decade who ditched it once they switched to a keto lifestyle. I didn't ask them to stop the ibuprofen. Instead, they became relatively pain-free about 6 weeks after they made the keto switch.

RINGING IN EARS

Tinnitus is the fancy term for ringing in the ears. Tinnitus is almost always linked to chronic inflammation within the ear. I have spent hundreds of hours helping patients with this condition. Patients suffer from a constant buzzing in their ears-without escape. The buzzing is caused by the presence of extra water molecules inside the delicate inner parts of their ear. The water does not belong there, yet it is trapped in a cycle of inflammation.

I recommended the ketosis diet to a patient of mine who was suffering from Parkinson's disease. She was about eighty pounds overweight and also suffered from chronic tinnitus. She asked for support from her granddaughter who was also trying to lose weight. To my surprise, it was not the twenty-five pounds of weight that she lost that excited her the most. Instead, she remarked repeatedly how the ringing in her ears disappeared nearly two months after going keto. Because this medical problem is such a lonely and trying ordeal-much like a personal prison, I reached out to two other patients and suggested a ketone-producing diet. Both of these chronic sufferers agreed to transition into ketosis for a minimum of three months. At their 90-day follow up, one had complete resolution of her tinnitus and the other said he had several days in a row without the noise-something he had not experienced in over five years.

Although this is not a formal study looking into a connection between ketosis and tinnitus, the difference this advice made in the lives of these patients is priceless. I contend tinnitus is one of many chronic nagging symptoms of long-term inflammation.

When you use fat for your body's energy source and stop consuming carbs, swelling disappears because there is no longer an abundance of glucose molecules holding onto extra water. At first, the easiest swelling goes away, like that in your blood vessels and your muscles. The longer you stay in ketosis, the better your body drains chronic inflammation re-solving tinnitus.

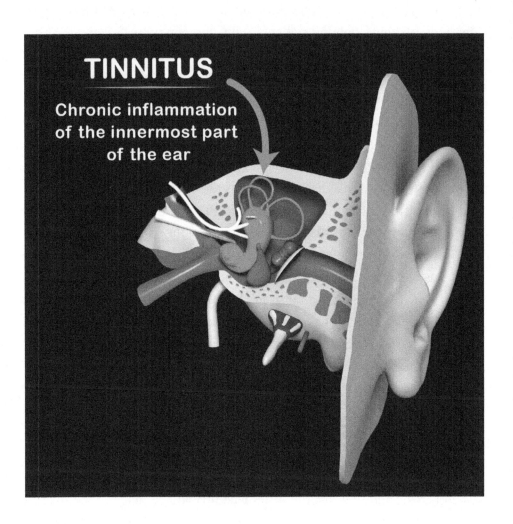

GINGIVITIS / HALITOSIS

Gingivitis occurs when the gums lining each of your teeth swell. Halitosis means bad breath. I talk about these together because they are closely linked. Patients with chronic sensitive teeth or gum disease tell me that producing ketones helped improve their oral health.

At first, keto patients report bad breath. Part of this is due to the acetone-a byproduct of ketosis -they are breathing out. The change in your breath also reflects the dramatic shift in your mouth's bacteria. Prior to ketones, the bacteria inside the mouth and in the saliva use glucose and other sugars as their main energy source. After the switch, these bugs die off because they no longer have the fuel they need to live. The death of sugar-hungry bacteria reduces swelling in your gums and the smell in your breath.

The cells in a keto-adapted mouth compared to someone with swollen gums are much like the improved skin cells I mentioned earlier. The keto-adapted cells are plumper, more flexible, and fit together tighter. This is protective against the roots of your teeth.

PAINKILLERS / ANTI-INFLAMMATORY

When helping patients deal with pain, I can always pull out the big hammer of narcotics like morphine or Oxycontin. But this hammer comes with the very serious drawback of addiction. More often, physicians like to prescribe anti-inflammatories. The most intense of these are steroids. When comparing steroids to other compounds, these remove inflammation the best.

While doctors like the power of using a steroid medication to dissipate inflammation, these chemicals carry significant risks when used long term. Instead, we'll use a non-steroid anti-inflammatory. This is abbreviated as NSAID--Non-Steroidal Anti-Inflammatory Drugs such as ibuprofen or naproxen. These are safe enough to buy over the counter, yet aren't as great at reducing inflammation when compared to steroids. In fact, we estimate steroid-medications as ten times more effective in knocking out inflammation over non-steroids.

By way of comparison, when I instruct someone to take ibuprofen for an ache or a pain, I teach them that the medication will help their pain for eight hours. When setting expectations about how much improvement they should expect, I tell them it's like a nickel. Yep - a nickel. They can use that ibuprofen every eight hours and expect a nickel's worth of improvement. If they need more help than ibuprofen can deliver, we prescribe the steroid such as prednisone. Prednisone lasts for twenty-four hours and it's worth fifty cents. Yep, it is ten times more powerful than the ibuprofen and you only take it once a day. If you take that prednisone several days in a row, it actually increases in value. The first day it helps the inflammation by fifty cents. The second day it helps a little more, about fifty-two cents. If you stack prednisone day after day the power to reduce inflammation keeps rising until about day 10. After that, it steadily sinks back to about twenty-five cents. The daily use of steroids also weakens your bones, thins your skin, increases your sugars, messes up your mood, and destroys your metabolism.

The moral of this story is that ibuprofen is a safe, yet mild anti-inflammatory. Prescription steroids are much more powerful, but after time they lose much of their power and have heavy consequences if used long term.

Interestingly enough, ketones are estimated to be ten times more powerful than steroid medications. Produce ketones for a month and the anti-inflammatory effect is worth $5.00!! Let's put it this way, going keto is 100 times more effective in reducing inflammation than using ibuprofen! Produce ketones for a year and it is estimated that it is worth $25.00!!

How is this possible?

When your body has excess water, your cells get inflamed. They balloon up. On a carb-heavy diet, your system fills up with lots of water molecules. The carb-derived glucose molecules in your system naturally grab onto water molecules. Just how much water are we talking about here? Hundreds of water molecules per glucose molecule! That's a lot of water. No wonder, arthritis sufferers on carb-rich diets get nasty inflammation attacks.

When your system stops carrying around extra glucose, it let's go of the water too. Remove that water in someone with arthritis and their joints hurt less. Stiffness is reduced.

Additionally, steroids are naturally made within your body. Steroid prescriptions remove inflammation because they mimic the steroids your body produces. Cortisol is one of your self-made-steroid hormones that removes inflammation. Your cortisol hormones began as fat. Nutritional ketosis boosts hormone production overall. Sustained ketosis improves your body's production of fat-based hormones across the board, including testosterone, estrogen, *cortisol,* and aldosterone.

MIGRAINE HEADACHES

Migraines suck. Not only do they ruin the day that they happen, but they also kill brain cells. That is not an exaggeration. When a severe, throbbing pain lasts for several hours, swollen brain cells die. Migraines cause brain damage by disrupting blood flow, much like a mini-stroke. Repeated disruption in brain blood flow kills more brain cells. Stop doing that at all costs-especially if you are a chronic migraine patient. I have yet to see a patient walk into my clinic and say, "I want to be on the ketosis diet because I heard it helps with migraines." However, I hope this book brings some of them in. Teaching patients to produce ketones has become the most effective way to get my patients off of migraine medication and on to a healthy pain-free life. The root reason is the anti-inflammatory effects of ketosis.

Just like other chronic problems, migraines don't cause brain damage overnight. Similarly, recovering from years of swollen and damaged tissue takes time. The authentic migraine antidote starts when the patient becomes fully keto-adapted, about 4-6 weeks into the production of ketones. As they continue to practice the lifestyle and take it to higher and higher levels, we see patients reporting a complete end to their migraines-usually within 6 months of peeing on that first ketone stick.

The longer you stay in ketosis, the more completely you remove the amount of extra brain swelling water. At first, the easy water gets shed from the swelling in your legs and bloating in your gut. Over the next few months, you'll also experience water removal in your skin, joints, eyes, and brain. You can't help but observe the following: glowing skin, better joint movements, reduced neck pain, and improved eyesight. These positive improvements show up around the 3-6 month mark, precisely the time most patients' migraines disappear.

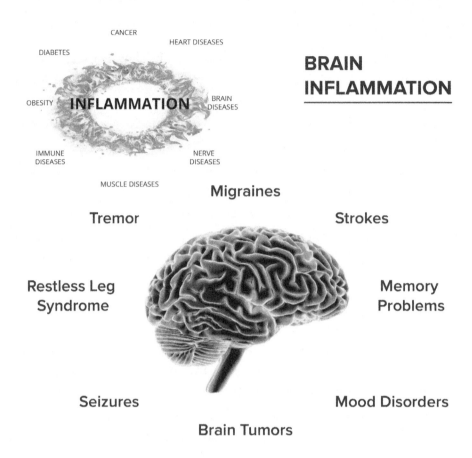

BRAIN INFLAMMATION

OBJECTION #3: "Low carb causes depression. My friend did it and totally got depressed."

Certainly, I have seen the depression, lethargy, and tiredness that happened when patients transition from a heavy carb diet to a low carb diet. Just as often, I see some patients struggle with a rise in anger and anxiety when they transition. Switching fuel sources from carbs to fat affects all areas of the body-especially the brain. That striking change is FOR THE BETTER. The transition is tough. I'm not going to lie. The good news? There are tools to help you get through the switch as quickly and successfully as possible.

When people are tired, irritable, and have brain fog, they come to see me. Or their family drags them in on a stretcher. After we rule out the dangerous, life-threatening problems, often their brain funk is traced back to sugar.

TASTE

Plan on a burst in flavor from your food. Maybe this comes from the improved dopamine produced by a well-nourished brain. Or maybe from the well-needed reset after years of constantly flooding your taste-buds with sweeteners.

Strangely, patients report this even as they eat less and less food! The natural tendency to eat less when fueling the body with fat happens in every patient. Once their hunger fades, it only takes a minor coaxing to help them recognize the difference between eating because the clock says so versus eating due to actual hunger.

Once they let go of the eat-according-to-the-clock tradition, many of my ketosis patients eat only one meal a day. Despite their lower eating frequency, patient after patient shared their intensely rewarding eating experiences.

Chapter 9
Grandma Rose: THE VERDICT

We arrived at the cancer doctor's office two hours early for a new round of blood tests. The nurse drew Grandma Rose's blood sample. We then sat silently waiting for the results.

I thought about the other times when Grandma Rose needed chemotherapy-once in 2010 and another in 2013.

This time around, things were different. Sure, she was older, but as we sat there, she didn't look as sick. The last time we sat there, she looked hollow. She had been battling against one infection after another. Those constant infections strapped her like thousands of strands of dental floss pulling her down. Each individual infection held a small amount of power. When they occurred together, they packed a knockout punch that was simply too much-even for Mary Poppins.

Before CLL, she blocked those invading infections easily, but her CLL kept chipping away at Mary Poppins. When her CLL took five months to double, she needed antibiotics two weeks out of four. Then it grew faster and doubled in six weeks. She could not go off of the antibiotics until chemo reduced her cancer load. Both times, the treatment was harsh.

Each cycle of chemo ended with improved laboratory results. All her scores looked better after the chemo but the journey transformed her into an older, weaker, less-resilient version of Grandma Rose.

My mind danced back and forth wondering if Grandma Rose would need chemo again. The numbers would make the decision.

Had they doubled in the past six weeks? Tripled?

I remembered her ashen look the last time we awaited to hear if chemo was needed. A gray shadow lurked under her skin and whispered the worry of death. No shadow was there that day. Maybe my mind played tricks on me to draw me away from the worry.

Even if chemo was just around the corner, she was certainly healthier somehow. Six weeks ago she made her first ketone, and it dawned on me in that waiting room that she had not needed antibiotics in the last 5 weeks. Coincidence? Or evidence?

I was prepared for today-whatever it might bring. Maybe our bond had strengthened further as we tackled this strange diet together. Something told me that she was stronger this time around.

Finally, the doctor arrived.

It was unlike him to run this late. He sat on his stool and asked his usual questions. His voice had an unmistakable tone of curiosity. It made me nervous.

"I am running a bit behind because I called the lab and asked them to re-run the numbers today. You both know that CLL does not get better with time. It speeds up over time. Six weeks ago, your numbers had doubled in just two months. Today, the numbers have not doubled. They have not increased by even 50%. They haven't even increased by 10%."

"They have decreased by thirty percent!"

Shocked into tears, our excitement warned the doctor of something suspicious.

"This never happens. What have you been doing?"

Wide-eyed, we both shot each other the same look and said nothing.

He waited in suspense. We waited hoping he would just keep going on with his busy doctor-filled day.

He paused longer.

Together, we lied, "Nothing."

We left Mary Poppins' high moral ground and just straight out lied to the doctor. He wasn't fooled.

He smiled and said, "Whatever you're doing, keep it up. I'll see you again in three months."

Chapter 10

Lessons from Dr. Bosworth:

FRUIT IS EVIL

If you hate science and math, skip this chapter. Yes, that's right. Just read the title, believe it … and move on to the next chapter.

For the rest of you, I will prove to you mathematically that fruit is evil.

Let's begin with an ancient story where man was tempted by the evils of fruit. Yes, I'm talking about Adam and Eve and the tree with the forbidden fruit. From the beginning of time, we've heard stories of Satan being associated with fruit.

Well, that story lives on. Marketers taught my generation and several before mine that fruits are essential to living. This simply is not true. Don't get me wrong, like most sins, there's a sweet, juicy, heavenly high that comes after a wonderful piece of fruit. Still, the math of your body chemistry proves that fruit is evil.

Let's begin with a little experiment on your body.

Step 1) Go to your cupboard and find one of the most sugar-rich, sweetest substances you can. Look at the label, find the highest content of carbohydrates or sugars you can. Might I suggest a jar of jam, honey, or a stash of your favorite candy bar?

Step 2) Eat 2 cups full of that food right now. Your pine needle fire will start to burn in as little as 10 minutes. Your blood sugar will shoot up like a rocket.

Step 3) Right before your rising sugar triggers your insulin to squirt from your pancreas, prick your finger to get a drop of blood. Let's say that drop of blood measured your glucose level at 100 milligrams per deciliter. Your blood sugar was 100 mg/dl.

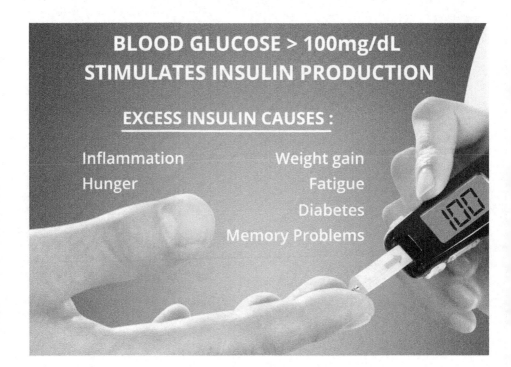

BLOOD GLUCOSE > 100mg/dL STIMULATES INSULIN PRODUCTION

EXCESS INSULIN CAUSES :

Inflammation   Weight gain
Hunger   Fatigue
     Diabetes
     Memory Problems

Step 4) Next, drain all the blood from your body so that we can measure your volume of blood.

Okay, okay, I am getting carried away. For your safety, we will estimate the total volume of blood held inside all the arteries and veins in your body. Most people's complete blood supply ranges from five to seven liters.

We pricked your finger and checked your blood glucose at just the right timing to find 100 milligrams of sugar in every deciliter of your blood. This is the moment right before your body triggers evil insulin.

Your body holds approximately seven liters of blood.

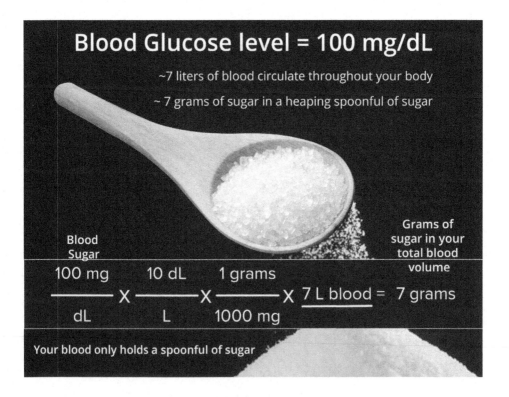

Blood Glucose level = 100 mg/dL

~7 liters of blood circulate throughout your body

~ 7 grams of sugar in a heaping spoonful of sugar

$$\frac{100 \text{ mg}}{\text{dL}} \times \frac{10 \text{ dL}}{\text{L}} \times \frac{1 \text{ grams}}{1000 \text{ mg}} \times \underline{7 \text{ L blood}} = 7 \text{ grams}$$

Blood Sugar

Grams of sugar in your total blood volume

Your blood only holds a spoonful of sugar

How many spoonfuls of sugar can be dissolved in your body before triggering insulin production? Remember, insulin is what KILLS ketone production.

Let's do the math. Look at this breakdown.

Think back to your 6th-grade algebra class. Convert all your labels back and forth with milligrams to grams and deciliters to liters. Your 7 liters of blood holds around 7 grams of sugar, otherwise known as a heaping teaspoon of sugar.

What the heck does this have to do with the evil spirit of fruit? Wait for it . . .
One teaspoon of sugar is just over 4 grams of carbohydrates.
A rounded teaspoon is 6-7 grams of carbs.

YOUR PANCREAS DOES NOT CARE if the carbohydrates came from cane sugar or from that fluffy piece of bread, or from applesauce. Your body will turn all those carbohydrates into sugars for your mitochondria to burn hot and fast.

Eat a slice of bread and add about 20 grams of carbohydrates or 5 heaping teaspoons of sugar to your bloodstream. That means one of those spoons of sugar found in that slice of bread will circulate into the bloodstream as glucose, but evil insulin will whip the other four spoons of sugar into storage pockets throughout your body.

Yep, insulin pushes those extra carbohydrates away into storage cells. Usually, these storage cells are your fat cells. And those stored carbs stay there-until you choose to pee ketones.

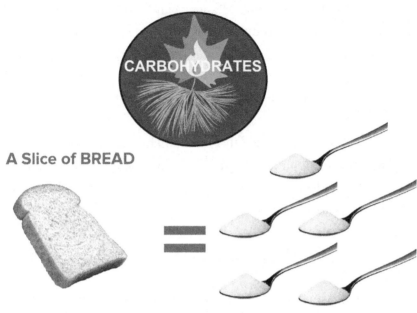

A Slice of BREAD

1 slice of bread = 5 spoons of sugar

Do you see why it can take some patients days to pee their first ketone? They have been storing sugar for years!

Play along. Go buy urine ketone strips. They're cheap-around $15 for 50 strips. You'll find them at your local drugstore. No doctor's prescription needed. Just tell the pharmacist you need urine ketone strips.

Don't change a stinkin' thing about the way that you fuel your body.

Now pee on one of those ketone sticks 3-4 times a day just to see if once, in a whole week, you turn on the ketone producing part of your body.

You'll know you're producing ketones if your strip turns pink. Even a hint of pink means you win.

Most likely, you won't produce any ketones. Most of my patients don't. They don't even know how.

Let's use another example. Take a bowl of rice. A little over a cup of rice contains 15 teaspoons of sugar. That's 60 grams of carbohydrates in it.

Switch to a bowl of pasta, and you have 20 teaspoons of sugar or 80 grams of carbohydrates.

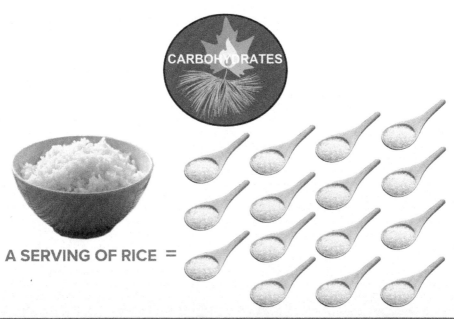

A SERVING OF RICE =

1 serving of rice = 15 spoons of sugar

Let's make the final step to close this loop. Take notice of the chart at the end of this chapter.

This is a list of fruits and the number of carbohydrates found in a 1/2 cup of each item. Look at the column to the far right. You'll see the grams of carbs each serving contains.

Remember, our leveled teaspoon of sugar held 4 grams of carbohydrates. If we rounded the teaspoon of sugar, it was closer to 5-7 grams of carbohydrates.

½ CUP OF FRUIT	CALORIES	FAT (grams)	CARBOHYDRATES (grams)
Apple	33	0	9
Avocado	120	11	6
Banana	67	0	17
Blueberries	42	0	11
Cantaloupe	27	0	11
Cherries	48	0	12
Fig, dried	186	1	48
Fig, fresh (1 large)	47	0	12
Grapefruit	38	0	10
Grapes	55	0	14
Guava	56	1	12
Honeydew	31	0	8
Kiwifruit	54	0	13
Kumquat (6 medium)	81	1	18
Lemon	31	0	10
Lime (1 medium)	20	0	7

½ CUP OF FRUIT	CALORIES	FAT (grams)	CARBOHYDRATES (grams)
Mango	54	0	14
Nectarine	31	0	8
Orange	42	0	11
Papaya	27	0	7
Peach	30	0	7
Pear	41	0	11
Pineapple	39	0	10
Plum	38	0	9
Plum, dried	204	0	54
Pomegranate (½ fruit)	52	0	13
Raisins (½ cup, packed)	247	0	65
Raspberries	32	0	7
Star Fruit	17	0	4
Strawberries	27	0	6
Tangerine	52	0	13
Watermelon	23	0	6

Line 1 - An apple-a half-cup of apple holds 9 grams of carbohydrates. Go look at the size of a half-cup. This will not fit a whole apple. A whole apple gives us somewhere between 18-25 carbohydrates.

Line 2 - Half a cup of a banana holds 17 carbs. Check out the dried fruit. Yikes! For years I have told patients and my kids to eat these for fiber.

Busted. My kids ate those raisins and their blood sugar shot up, sparking insulin production. Their bodies turned 4 of the 65 raisin carbs found in that ½ cup into pine needle-like energy. The other 61 were stuffed into storage in the form of fat.

Verdict? Fruit is evil.

Fruits have been sold to all of us as healthy and nourishing. The truth is the opposite. We've been sold a bill of goods. Fruits are filled with sugary carbohydrates.

Fruits hold no essential ingredient for life. They are treats that should only be eaten 3-4 times a year. The amount of sugar found in the fruits we eat today far exceeds what our bloodstream can hold. We shove that extra sugar into all sorts of nasty storage spaces in the name of 'healthy living.'

Excess sugar ages our body causes heart disease, and wilts our brains.

The solution? Fuel your body with ketones for a week.

You won't regret it.

Chapter 11

Lessons from Dr. Bosworth:
INSULIN RULES

I personally continue to fuel my body with ketones because of its effect on brain function. Ketosis' main attraction to most people is its ability to produce smooth, almost effortless weight loss.

Ketosis makes weight loss quicker and easier. In fact, losing weight on a keto diet is a 'no brainer' for many people. How come? It all boils down to insulin. Insulin opens and closes the gates of all of your fat cells.

If there's insulin near a fat storing cell, all fat stays locked inside. If you want to use the energy of your fat cells, insulin must leave the scene. Insulin is also the chemical messenger that allows glucose into the cell. Without insulin, those extra glucose molecules never gain access to your furnaces. They remain in your bloodstream, outside your cells.

Fat Loss and the Role of Insulin

When a patient asks for weight loss help, it often goes without saying that they are asking for help to get rid of their excess fat. No one has ever asked me to help them shed weight by trimming muscle tissue. Weight loss means getting rid of the contents stuffed in your fat-storing cells. These cells fall under the commanding leadership of a very powerful ruler: INSULIN. Keep in mind the following rules.

Rule #1: Insulin is King

Energy storage is controlled by insulin. Insulin is the king of hormones. If insulin is present, glucose molecules are evacuated from your blood.

'Be GONE!' Where do the glucose molecules go? One of two options:

1) GLUCOSE AS FUEL: Insulin siphons the glucose from the bloodstream to the inside of your cells. These cells can be in your brain, liver, muscles, skin, or any other tissue. All will use glucose for energy.

2) GLUCOSE AS STORAGE: Insulin triggers your storage cells to suction any extra glucose from your bloodstream and store them. Most glucose gets stored as fat. Insulin orders all nearby **fat** cells to lock all their exits. Insulin orders the fat cells to not release any new energy into the system.

Your fat cells do not care about the origin of glucose in your blood. They only follow the command of their mighty dictator, insulin. Two hours ago, you washed down an apple with some orange juice. Your blood sugar rose and insulin squirted into your system. Because of that insulin, any sugar found in your system will be suctioned out of the bloodstream and put into the nearest storage cell.

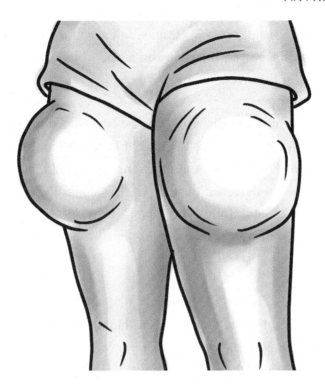

Fat cells cannot empty when insulin is around. You cannot use your stored fat as fuel as long as insulin is present.

This drawing is inspired by an old medical textbook picture showing a man whose body didn't produce any insulin. Thankfully, he lived during a time where injectable insulin was available.

I talk about insulin being evil. It is not all evil. It plays a necessary role in the healthy, normal operations of your body.

Your body needs a bare minimum of insulin to trade, store, and exchange energy. This hormone is needed for life. If you don't produce it, you're going to die young unless you inject it. This man has two large mounds of fatty tissue on each of his thighs.

He injected insulin into his thighs, in the same spots. Through the years, he injected insulin in the right thigh, then the left thigh-shot after shot after shot. Insulin saved his life.

He did not die from diabetes because he injected insulin. His pancreas failed to produce insulin. Notice what happened in those areas near the injection points? Fat grew. And grew and grew and grew. His thighs' muscle cells were not designed to store fat. But under the direction of insulin, his nearby fat cells followed orders. They turned on the vacuum and sucked glucose into storage. Those rounded mounds are over-stuffed fat cells.

The injection of insulin changed that area from predominantly muscle cells to all fat. His fat cells were hundreds of times larger than they're supposed to be because they were repeatedly influenced by doses of injected insulin. Over the course of several decades, insulin locked the fat inside those fat cells. He never went more than 24 hours without giving himself a shot. The fat that stored in those cells remained for decades. This next picture tells a similar story.

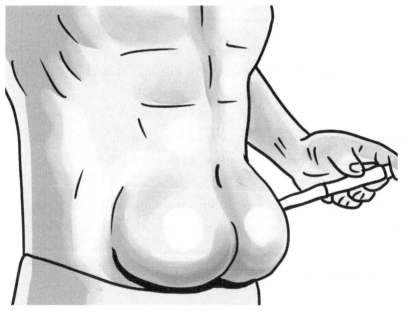

This patient injected insulin in the same two spots in his abdomen. Insulin commanded those cells to store fat. After many years of insulin injections, he chemically ordered those cells to overgrow and over-fill with fat.

This is a one-way door unless he runs out of insulin for several days. The only way he will release the fat from those cells is to stop instructing the storage of fat through the injection of insulin.

Before insulin injections became available, low carbohydrate diets kept Type 1 diabetics alive.

Here's an example of their recommended daily nutrient breakdown from 1915:

      10 grams of carbohydrates, 40 calories
      75 grams of protein, 300 calories
      150 grams fat, 1350 calories.
      15 grams of alcohol

Almost all their calories came from fat. I'm not quite sure why they added 15 grams of alcohol, but that was also in the diet. It was probably distilled alcohol which has no carbohydrates in it. Alcohol completely stops the production of ketones in the liver. Alcohol, like a ketone, enters your cells without insulin. Without insulin, no glucose enters the cells. Glucose <u>inside the cell</u> stops ketone production. Without insulin to carry the glucose inside their cells, these 1915 diabetics had no 'brakes' for their ketone production, except for alcohol. Alcohol's inclusion in their diet might have prevented ketoacidosis - that dangerous buildup of excess ketones in the body that can lead to coma and death.

QUANTITY OF FOOD Required by a Severe Diabetic Patient Weighing 60 kilograms, (Joslin.)

Food	Quantity Grams	Calories per Gram	Total Calories
Carbohydrate	10	4	40
Protein	75	7	300
Fat	150	9	1,350
Alcohol	15	7	105
			1,795

STRICT DIET. (Foods without sugar.) Meats, Poultry, Game, Fish, Clear Soups, Gelatine, Eggs, Butter, Olive Oil, Coffee, Tea and Cracked Cocoa.

FOOD ARRANGED APPROXIMATELY ACCORDING TO CONTENT OF CARBOHYDRATES

	5% ±		10% ±	15% ±	20% ±
VEGETABLES	Lettuce Spinach Sauerkraut String Beans Celery Asparagus Cucumbers Brussels Sprouts Sorrel Endive Dandelion Greens Swiss Chard Vegetable Marrow	Cauliflower Tomatoes Rhubarb Egg Plant Beet Greens Water Cress Cabbage Radishes Pumpkin Kohl-Rabi Son Kale	Onions Squash Turnip Carrots Okra Mushrooms Beets	Green Peas Artichokes Parsnips Canned Lima Beans	Potatoes Shell Beans Baked Beans Green Corn Boiled Rice Boiled Macaroni
FRUITS	Ripe Olives (20 per cent. Fat) Grape Fruit		Lemons Oranges Cranberries Strawberries Blackberries Gooseberries Peaches Pineapples Watermelon	Apples Pears Apricots Blueberries Cherries Currants Raspberries Huckleberries	Plums Bananas
NUTS	Butternuts Pignolias		Brazil Nuts Black Walnuts Hickory Pecans Filberts	Almonds Walnuts (Eng.) Beechnuts Pistachios Pine Nuts	Peanuts **40% ±** Chestnuts
Miscellaneous	Unsweetened and Unspiced Pickle Clams Oysters Scallops Liver Fish Roe				

Normally, insulin is secreted from your pancreas every time your guts sense carbohydrates. For example, milk has sugar in it called lactose. As soon as your gut detects that lactose, it triggers your pancreas to squeeze out some insulin. Insulin then permeates the body, and orders cells to vacuum up sugar out of the blood, causing your blood sugar level to drop. As insulin instructs your cells to soak up sugars. It also flows past fat cells. Insulin commands fat cells to lockdown their exits and suck in any extra nearby energy. Stored energy can't leave fat cells. The entrance doors to the fat cells still work; the exits don't.

If you want to empty your fat cells, you must turn off the vacuum pulling your energy into these cells. The on/off switch for your fat cells' vacuum is insulin. To empty your body's fat storage cells, stop making insulin.

How do you stop producing insulin? Stop eating carbohydrates.

Listed below are certain common foods and their impact on ketosis. If you want less fat insulating your body, stop making so much insulin. Less insulin means weight loss-specifically from your fat cells. The following fattening foods lock down your fat cells from releasing any of your stored fat.

FATTENING FOOD

Bread: Anything made from wheat flour, white flour, pumpernickel flour, rye flour, tortillas, waffles, rolls, pasta, raisin bread

Cereals and Grains: bran cereals, cooked cereals, stuffing, unsweetened cereals, cornmeal, couscous, granola, grape-nuts, grits, pasta, quinoa, rice, brown rice, shredded wheat, sugar cereals

Fruit Juices: All juices associated with fruit, except lemon or lime juice in small quantities.

Fruit: Apple, applesauce, dried apples, apricots, bananas, cantaloupe, cherries, grapefruit, grapes, Kiwi, honeydew, mangoes, mandarin oranges, nectarines, oranges, Papaya, Peaches, pears, pineapples, raisins, tangerines, dried fruit

Beans, Peas, and Nuts: baked beans, black beans, peas, garbanzo beans, pinto beans, kidney beans, white beans, split beans, black-eyed beans, lima beans, cashew nuts, chestnuts, tofu, soybeans

Milk: nonfat milk, chocolate milk, evaporated milk, skim milk, whole milk, soy milk, nonfat yogurt.

Bad Carb-Vegetables: corn, peas, potatoes, squash, yams, sweet potatoes

Snacks: animal crackers, goldfish crackers, graham crackers, oyster crackers, popped popcorn, pretzels, sandwich crackers, chips, tortilla chips, potato chips, french fries

Sweets: Anything with sugar, honey, or other sweeteners. Cake, biscuits, brownies, candy, chocolate, cookies, sauces, donuts, ice cream, jams, jellies, ketchup, pie, frosting

WEIGHT LOSS FOOD: Eat these for fat loss

Fat: Ironically enough, to lose flab, you need to eat fat. How come? There are no carbs found in fat. No insulin is produced when you consume fat. Just make sure not to add sugar (or other carbohydrates) to your fat.

MEAT: beef, pork, ham, lamb, veal, bacon, pork belly, or any game meat (rabbit, moose, elk, venison)
> **WARNING**: Excess protein trigger insulin production.

> **Processed Meat**: salami, pepperoni, sausage, Spam, liverwurst, bologna, hot dogs, bacon, ham. Make sure these are loaded with fat and not 'light' or 'lean' versions.

> **Poultry**: chicken, turkey, duck, pheasant or any game birds.
> > **Note**: Eat the skin. That's where most of the fat is. Looking for breading without carbs? Use pork rinds.

> **Seafood**: any fish or shellfish. Here is an incomplete list: salmon, halibut, cod, crab, prawns, clams, oysters, mussels, squid, octopus, smoked fish, dried fish, canned fish /seafood (sardines, tuna)

Eggs: Whole eggs. When in doubt, add more yolks.
> Allergic to eggs? Consult with your doctor about eating only the yolks. The protein in the egg white is where most egg allergies originate.

SALAD/ LEAVES: (range from 0.5–5 carbs per 1 cup) leafy greens, dandelion, beet greens, collards, mustard greens, turnip, arugula, chicory, endive, escarole, fennel, radicchio, romaine lettuce, sorrel, spinach, kale, chard, parsley, lettuce, onion tops, leeks, alfalfa sprouts, seaweed

Vegetables:

Cruciferous vegetables: (ranges 3–6 grams of carbs per 1 cup) Brussels sprouts, broccoli, cabbage, cauliflower, turnips, garden cress, watercress

Uncooked vegetables that grow above ground: (2–4 grams of carbs per 1 cup) Celery, cucumber, zucchini, chives, leeks, asparagus, eggplant

Uncooked vegetables higher in carbs- only in moderation: (3–7 grams of carbs per 1 cup) asparagus, mushrooms, bamboo shoots, bean sprouts, bell pepper, sugar snap peas, water chestnuts, radishes, jicama, green beans, wax beans, tomatoes

Cooked Vegetables: (15-25 grams of carbs per 1 cup-- **WARNING**: These vegetables throw most people out of ketosis.) Eat once every 6 weeks. Sweet peas, artichokes, okra, carrots, beets, and parsnips.

Don't go overboard with vegetables since they contain carbohydrates. Instead, think of them as nutritional 'vehicles' that carry fat to your guts. Add olive oil, sour cream, butter or other fats to your vegetables. Make sure you don't overcook them.

Cheese: Choose full-fat cheeses, not low-fat. The high-fat, hard cheeses have the fewest carbs.

Full-fat cheeses: (0.5–1.5 grams carbs per one ounce or about 1/4 cup) Gouda, Brie, Edam, Cheddar, Colby, goat cheese, Swiss

Aged cheeses: Cheddar, Gruyere, Manchego, Gouda and Parmesan (Parmigiano-Reggiano / Grana Padano Such)

Soft Cheeses: Camembert, Brie, blue, feta, Swiss, goat cheese, Monterey jack, mozzarella

Dairy: Heavy whipping cream, sour cream

If you want to empty your fat cells, change your body's chemistry to unlock the exit doors. Decrease the insulin first. Insulin blocks weight loss.

.

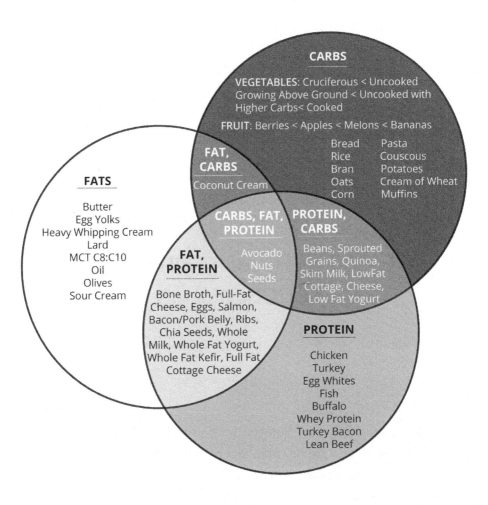

Chapter 12

Grandma Rose: AT FIRST WE SUCCEEDED ...

"Whatever you're doing, keep it up. I'll see you again in three months."

We did that? Was that us?

Had six weeks of ketosis reversed Grandma Rose's cancer growth? Ketosis decreased her numbers by 30%?

The doctor in me said, "No way."

Yet, one look at her and my inner skeptic was stunned. My eyes took in a woman snatched from the past and brought to the here and now as if through time travel.

I had not considered the option that her numbers would decrease. I hoped and prayed for them not to increase as much, but never once considered they could decrease.

We claimed the success and celebrated with chocolate keto fat bombs. Our days of eating heavy whipping cream, checking ketones and avoiding carbs had paid off. We were genuinely proud. Grateful. We had changed the course of her cancer.

My joy soon faded to anger. Why did no one else know about this? Why isn't the universe recommending this to all cancer patients?

It was my fault. I am in the prime of my career as an Internal Medicine physician. Why did it take the near-death of my mother for me to learn about this? Sadly, I caught the idea in the hushed voice of my patient. My curiosity grew after hearing more about ketosis from a podcast instead of a medical journal or a public service announcement.

'Do or Die.'

When facing death, our focus and discipline produced a perfect scorecard. But like with any change in habits, our success at reaching that short-term goal left us a little lost the first week after her appointment. Saying you are going to do keto forever is one thing, especially if 'forever' is only six weeks away. Sticking to a keto lifestyle indefinitely is another matter entirely. We faced some struggles.

Take the example of beer. We'd both given up beer during that initial crunch time. It wasn't a big sacrifice when we only looked ahead for six weeks. On our countdown to the big check-up, we were strictly alcohol-free. Greatly motivated by the threat of cancer, neither of us was willing to sacrifice one day out of ketosis for a silly beer. But now that we found ourselves on the other side of our goal, a beer sounded like an okay idea again.

One single beer took me out of ketosis. Zilch. No ketones.

I expected an instant return of ketones after that beer experiment. Instead, three days passed before my ketone strip turned pink again. Strange.

Why? Reading through the rules and literature, I learned that distilled liquors like tequila, or rum, or gin contained no carbohydrates.

It turned out neither of us tolerated such 'hard' drinks. Those types of alcohol sparked a headache each morning after we tried the distilled liquors. Drinking concentrated alcohol inflamed Grandma Rose's brain so much that her migraines from decades ago returned.

With beer off the list and hard liquors too intense for either of us, we turned to red wine. Have you ever tried to look at the carbohydrates in a glass of wine? Yeah, it wasn't there. Nobody cared how many carbs were in your glass of wine.

I wasn't the first person to run into this problem. When it comes to wines, the sweeter the wine, the higher the carbohydrates. The dryer the wine, the lower the carbohydrates. This also correlates with the pH or acid-base ratio of the wine.

We fully explored this diversion when we walked into a liquor store and asked the attendant to show us the lowest carbohydrate wine they sold.

Yep, the attendant was clueless.

We shifted gears and asked about their 'driest' wines. No such luck either. They took a guess. We bought their recommendation of a so-called, 'dry' wine and each drank a glass. Neither of us made ketones for two days. Bugger.

DRY FARM WINES: If you want a solution to the low carbohydrate wine puzzle, check this company out. Dry Farm Wines tests wines for their dryness. They look at the sugar or carbohydrate content for each specific batch of wine. Don't let that word 'dry' confuse you into thinking it's alcohol-free wine. No, this company caters to the ketosis market by testing wines' carbohydrate levels. Once they have identified a low-carbohydrate wine, they broker it to people who are looking to stay in ketosis and still enjoy a glass of wine.

Two months after our positive report from the oncologist, Grandma and I both found ourselves slacking quite a bit on keto rules. Both of us stopped checking for ketones as often. We told ourselves that we could both feel when we were in ketosis. That was only partly true.

Without our 'do or die' goal in front of us, it's easy to lie. Just tell yourself the truth you want. When I wasn't checking for ketones, I would convince myself that it was okay that I didn't check. It was okay that I sometimes didn't achieve ketosis because we reached that goal previously.

We also struggled with our use of sugar substitutes: stevia, xylitol, Truvia, erythritol and so on. When starting out on my ketosis lifestyle, my craving for sweets seemed almost irresistible.

My medical degree did not protect me from wanting that serving of evening carbohydrates. This old habit of eating comfort snacks every evening wrecked my plan. My family has a late night ice cream bowl custom that transcends generations. Additionally, I could mindlessly eat 3 cups of 'healthy' macadamia nuts. Who does that?

Apparently, I did when my default carb-comforts were thrown out. Despite macadamia nuts being on the 'really good for you' keto list, I had to stop buying them. I could not resist the temptation once I started.

Determined not to fail, we found several recipes that used cacao powder, or peanut butter powder with heavy whipping cream plus one of the sugar substitutes. These recipes filled with high fat and sugar substitutes are called 'fat bombs' in the keto world. They were all 'safe.' We would still pee ketones the next morning, and that was good enough for us.

One night, my extreme sugar substitute use reached a toxic level. I had a particularly stressful day and indulged my sweet tooth in the name of therapy. I strategically removed all of my high-carb options for exactly this reason. When I got irritable and wanted sugar, please PLEASE don't put it within arms reach of me. I might bite your hand off.

There I was in the middle of the kitchen-all irritable, crabby, and just wanting some instant comfort thanks to sugar. I started pulling things out of the cupboard to make a favorite comforting recipe. It called for 3 cups of sugar mixed with half as much flour. I googled how to convert the recipe into a keto-ish recipe. I used almond flour plus coconut flour instead of the wheat flour. Then I calculated how to substitute erythritol for the three cups of sugar.

I mixed it up and put it into the oven. Forty minutes later, out came the best-smelling memory.

I prepared some whipped cream with even more erythritol. I invited the family to join me in my misery. They all stopped eating after a couple of bites. Not me. I ate three pieces.

I went to bed feeling only a little bit ashamed for how far I took that sugar craving. Whatever guilt or shame I suppressed arose out of my guts at two o'clock in the morning. I launched out of bed barely making it to the toilet. Every bite of that science experiment exploded from my backside for the rest of the night. The party inside my guts haunted me well into the next day as punishment for my sugar binge. Bloated, swollen, and filled with enough gas to power a small city, I vowed not to do that again.

On the eighth week after Grandma Rose's last oncologist appointment, I found myself using more and more sugar substitutes. Unlike my initial diarrhea explosion, their effect wasn't as nasty when I gradually increased the dose of sugar substitutes. Still, their sweet taste would ignite my cravings for more sugar or sweetness. My resistance to sugar began to crumble.

Chapter 13

Lessons from Dr. Bosworth:

LET'S BEGIN YOUR KETO JOURNEY

Step 1: No sugar. No starch. High fat.

The best summary of this diet is "no sugar, no starch, high fat." Say those words out loud. Again. No sugar. No starch. High fat.

Step 2: Remember the Number 20

This is really important as I will explain later. For now, commit this number to memory: 20

Step 3: Buy Urine Ketone Strips

I hate to even have to say this, but I recommend you buy something. Yes, as a physician who has been subjected to more multi-level marketing pitches than I care to admit, typing this recommendation makes me uncomfortable. But it is absolutely necessary.

To succeed at switching your fuel source from sugar to fat, you need to know if you are producing ketones. Spend some money. Ketone strips typically cost about $15. Purchase the smallest quantity you can. I buy bottles of 50 strips. I have put them in every single bathroom at my clinic and my house. I have even been known to leave a bottle at a friend's house because she constantly complained that she could not lose weight.

This is super important because the keto diet is measurable! This is my favorite part.

I have coached patients for decades that come in and say "Doctor, doctor, my diet is just not working for me." And they're right. The scale didn't move…

These changes seem strange to most everyone I advise. Keto strips allow me to measure patients' compliance. More importantly, the strips allow patients themselves to monitor their progress.

In the first two weeks, I want you peeing ketones as quickly as possible. Burning fat for fuel is the basis of this diet. Getting to the other side has proven to be unique to each patient. You will need the feedback that what you're doing in YOUR SPECIFIC situation is the right thing for you.

Some patients, usually men, stumble into ketosis. They pee ketones within 24 hours of changing habits. They may not always stay there but they can pee a ketone mighty quickly.

Other patients may take several weeks to burn through their stored sugar and struggle with their body chemistry due to insulin resistance.

Sometimes this is because they don't know what they're doing. But more often than not, their bodies were simply locked into using only sugar for fuel for years - if not decades. Some have been living with chronically high insulin levels for years. It can take weeks to burn up all the extra stored glucose in the body and finally see their insulin fall back to normal range. Remember, you can't produce ketones until both your blood sugar and your insulin comes down.

How resistant is your body to insulin?

There is a blood test you can take to get the answer. I offer this to my patients when I see them in the clinic, but I don't routinely recommend it. The test is expensive and coupled with the cost of a doctor's visit. It won't tell you anything you don't already know-you are addicted to sugar and have been for a long time. You have gained weight and can't seem to lose it because of your body's insulin cycle.

You will have a rotten time giving up carbs initially. Most people don't need a blood test to tell them that. Spend your efforts and money measuring something that does matter: The time it took for you to start producing ketones. Start using those urine sticks! If they turn pink, this means you made ketones. Pat yourself on the back, jot down how long it took you to pee that first ketone-and keep going!

Step 3.5: Buy MCT C8:C10

We will get into how to use this powdered fat supplement later. For now, just click on BUY and get it shipped to your home. Local stores are not likely to have this on hand, so I recommend searching the internet for direct delivery. Search these words: MCT C8:C10

Step 4: Empty Your Cupboards

This is a huge step. Empty out your cupboards.

One of the hardest changes you will have to make when adjusting to a high fat, low-carb diet is dealing with temptations. You need to put a lot of distance between yourself and the high carb foods you previously loved to eat. Do yourself a big favor and rid your home completely of these distractions and temptations. Cleanse the places you control. When walking addicts through a recovery plan, we start by asking a friend to help them cleanse their environments. This means throwing away all the signals that tempt you to go back to your old habits.

For an alcoholic, this means booze bottles stashed in the silliest places. For a drug addict, it involves needles, spoons and lighters. For a carb addict, your enemy is processed food. The more food has been processed, the quicker it ends up in your mouth. Moments later, your system is crammed with glucose molecules ruining your ketosis. Insulin surges and ketone production stops.

Even when you have cleansed the areas you control, be prepared for temptation. The devil has placed carbohydrates everywhere-from gas stations to coffee shops to your workplace. Protect the sanctuary of your home. Keep carbs out.

How do you know which food items to throw away when rifling through your cupboard?

Look at each item's label. Any item with a high level of carbohydrates or sugars needs to go. When trying to decide to keep or throw something, another rule-of-thumb centers around processing. If the food is highly processed, lose it. In our family, we took a box and everything that was made with flour, rice, corn or had sugar in it, we simply put in the box and took to the community food pantry. This was therapeutic for my household. My kids helped with this. If they considered keeping it, I had them count how many ingredients were in the product. If it had more than 8 ingredients, we tossed it.

This can be very stressful. Do this with a friend and make sure you don't quit until it's done.

Here are just a few things that ended up in the box that we took to the food pantry:

Hamburger Helper

Bags of pasta

Bags of rice

Flour

Sugar

Refried beans

Cans of corn

Cans of pears and other fruits (remember, fruit is evil)

Ketchup

Step 5: PAUSE

After the cupboards are bare, STOP. PAUSE. Do not rush the next steps. Grocery shopping will still be there tomorrow. Just pause long enough to understand these next few steps.

I can't say this enough ... P.A.U.S.E.

Step 6: Remember That Number?

What was that number you were supposed to remember?
Yep: Twenty. 20.

To start on your path to ketosis, you are allowed 20 grams of carbohydrates per day.

The only thing I want you counting in a day is carbohydrates. Not calories. Not grams of fiber or fat or protein. Not pounds or inches. I only want you focused on carbohydrate grams.

Forget about net carbs. Forget about dietary fiber. Don't distract yourself with 'sugars.' Just remember 20 and start counting carbohydrates! Restrict yourself to only 20 carbohydrate grams per day.

Transitioning people's behaviors starts with clear instructions and something measurable.

The clear instructions?
20 grams of carbohydrates per day.

The measurable factor?
Peeing ketones.

Here's an objection I usually get when I discuss this step with my patients:

OBJECTION # 4: "Doc, calories matter. Why aren't you telling us to count calories?"

For the last four decades, the medical establishment in the US has been preaching that calories matter. The truth? They don't matter when insulin is ruling your body. We can talk about calorie balance after you're keto-adapted. But the first thing you need to focus on is reducing your bloodstream insulin level, and that means HIGH FAT, LOW CARB. Your mission right now is to get rid of those carbohydrates!

Step 7: Eat Enough Fat to Feel Full

This is what sets this diet apart-there is no starvation! There is no want for food. I'm not exaggerating. With this approach, there's enough fat feeding your body that you don't feel hunger. Your brain receives a powerful chemical message of fullness from your system. This process begins when you eat fat after cutting out sugar or carbs.

Don't believe me? You have my permission to begin your day tomorrow by eating a stick of butter. Yep. You read that correctly. After not eating anything for several hours (because you were asleep) you can have a stick of butter for breakfast. Add salt for added taste if you like. Pair it with water or black coffee. Still, the only 'food' you should eat is butter. Don't imagine this story. Do it. Listen carefully to what your body is saying. Notice the sensation your brain sends to your body? Your brain detects the signal that you are full when fat fills your stomach.

No wonder so many of my patients boast about how sustainable and satisfying the ketogenic diet is.

Step 8: Eat Only When You Are Hungry

Do not sabotage your system's chemical transition from sugar to fat by snacking unnecessarily.

Your habits may seem so automatic that you hardly become aware that you're snacking until the bag is empty. Recognize these habits. Bring the habit out of your subconscious by keeping a food log.

My downfall was morning breakfast. For so long I told myself that breakfast was the most important meal of the day. I did not stop to ask myself if I was really hungry or just eating breakfast out of habit. After two months of keto eating, I challenged myself: No calories until I felt hungry. When hunger hit, I would take in my favorite foods first: coffee with heavy whipping cream. Before long I stopped eating breakfast and sipped on my favorite coffee with cream until well into the afternoon.

If you're suffering from anxiety or stress, make sure you only eat when you're hungry instead of eating for comfort. If you do choose to snack, eat fat instead of carbs.

Step 9: Restrict Protein

Nearly every person I have coached at some point overate protein. They are confusing boosting fats with loading up on protein. Perfectly understandable. The notion of a high protein diet as a healthy option has been around for a long time. Bodybuilders and health food promoters all have a protein supplement to help you remain healthy. In our minds, it all seems natural that protein is healthy. Those same people think high fat diets are unnatural. According to this 'conventional wisdom,' it is safe to eat lots of protein and it is unhealthy to load up on fat.

What's going on here? Lipophobia: the fear of fat. The media won this game. They successfully frightened us from enjoying fat.

I correct this thinking by educating patients that we are solving a human biochemistry puzzle. Our body's chemistry controls weight loss. The most important piece in the puzzle is insulin. Keep insulin down, and weight loss happens.

In the absence of carbohydrates, fat does not spike your insulin. Fat also sends a strong hormonal message to your brain to stop eating. This chemical shift is what makes the keto diet so powerful and effective. Fat does not spike insulin. Carbs spike insulin. Excess protein spikes insulin, too. For me, the most difficult pantry item to throw away was the protein powder.

On a ketogenic diet, how much protein does it take to spike your insulin?

Here's the formula I teach my patients: write down your ideal body weight-the weight you want to be. I'm 5'3" and would love to be 125 lbs. again. Divide 125 (your ideal body weight in pounds) by 2.2. This is the highest number of protein grams per day that you should eat.

In my case that is about 56 grams of protein per day. It's okay to eat less than that, but don't overshoot that number. If I stay under that goal for the day, my insulin does not surge. The first month when I failed and failed and failed to produce my first ketone, I was adding a scoop of protein powder to heavy whipping cream. That one scoop had 50 grams of protein and blocked my insulin from falling. No ketosis.

The number 20 was the only number you need to remember-I insist you stick to that for now. This protein number only surfaces when patients are having trouble. If you are in week 2 and you still haven't peed ketones, you have a problem. The culprit? You're probably eating a high protein diet instead of a high fat one. This is the most common mistake I see.

Eat too many proteins and your body will start to squirt out insulin. Insulin is the enemy of ketones.

Chapter 14

Lessons from Dr. Bosworth:

KETONE SUCCESS = REGULAR KETONE CHECKS

Measure your ketones. It's what separates this lifestyle from the last fifteen attempts you had to improve your health. People fail when changing habits without accurate, real-time feedback. Ketones are unique. You don't accidentally start making ketones. Measure them. Prove to yourself (and your doctor) that you modified your lifestyle enough to make ketones.

How to Measure Ketones

There are three ways to check if you're producing ketones: blood, urine, and breath. These tests check for three types of molecules: Aceto-Acetate, Beta-Hydroxybutyrate, and Acetone.

Two of these chemicals are energy sources or fuel for your body: AcetoAcetate and Beta-HydroxyButyrate. Your body produces acetone as a byproduct as it processes ketones.

OBJECTION #5: "Isn't this the diet where your body gets so whacked out that you start producing fingernail polish remover?"

This objection truly made me laugh. But, the question does hold some truth. The question accurately references ACETONE as the compound that you breathe out when in nutritional ketosis.

Fuel your body with fat, and you produce ketones. Most Americans haven't produced ketones in a long time. Maybe that one time just after their 50th birthday when they celebrated with a screening colonoscopy. When patients drop carbs and eat mostly fat, their mitochondria begin to churn out ketones. The presence of ketones after years of eating high carbs pushes their body to 'remember' how to use fat-based energy. While your system adapts, extra ketones circulate. Your bloodstream holds quite a bit of extra ketones. Produce more ketones than your body can use at once, and your body gets rid of the extra.

You can pee them out.
You can breathe them out.
You can even sweat them out.

Acetoacetate, abbreviated AcAc, is the name of the extra ketones wasted in your urine. In your breath, the AcAc ketone breaks down further to acetone.

Yes, THAT Acetone-the same chemical found in fingernail polish remover. Breath-borne acetone does validate this urban myth-minus all the drama.

Acetoacetate (AcAc)

This ketone is one of the two ketones found in the blood. It is made inside your liver cell's mitochondria. AcetoAcetate exits liver cells and enters into your circulation to fuel other cells looking for energy. After weeks of making ketones, nearly every cell in your body will be trained to use it for energy. This state is called keto-adaptation. When your liver gets busy making fuel from fat, you can find too much of this compound in your bloodstream. When it gets too high, your body needs to do something.

An overabundance of ketones in the bloodstream is dangerous and your body has protections built in to not allow that. Your body has several ways to eliminate the excess ketones from your system before they create a toxic, acidic, biochemical mess called ketoacidosis.

One option is to remove acetoacetate through your urine. When you pee on ketone urine strips turning them pink, AcetoAcetate causes that chemical reaction. Whenever I see my ketone urine strip turn positive, I remind myself that these are extra calories that I just peed out. The weight loss headline should read, 'Ketosis: Pee Out Those Extra Fat Calories.'

Beta-hydroxybutyrate (BHB)

Like AcAc, this ketone is a fuel that circulates in your blood. It also travels from liver cells to other cells' mitochondria. Once in the furnaces, BHB is converted into energy. Ketone blood tests measure the amount of this compound in your circulation. This is the most accurate measurement of nutritional ketosis.

Acetone

Not a fuel. Acetone is a waste product made from excess acetoacetate, AcAc, in the bloodstream. Acetone escapes from the body through our breath.

Which is the best way to measure your ketones? Urine, blood, or breath?

URINE

I tell all patients to start with urine strips. These strips are cheap and portable. They are quite reliable when first transitioning from glucose to ketones. For the first several weeks, this is all I recommend. Personally, I used this approach for over six months before I splurged on a blood testing kit.

How come? In the first few weeks of any behavior change, beware of your past patterns.

Choose anything you have tried to change: smoking, drinking, better sleeping habits, exercising, dealing with an annoying coworker …

The biggest threat to your changed behavior comes from your past habits. The behavior change sticks around for awhile, but when stress or boredom strikes, your old ways show up again. Before long, your new habit has all but disappeared. Given this reality, I want patients to be on the lookout for their past habits.

How do you help someone become aware of something that seems automatic? Check urine ketones to be certain you are avoiding old patterns. Checking urine ketones is a painless, cheap, and portable way to stay accountable. Verify your ketone state by placing a few urine ketone strips in your pocket at the start of each day. Make this a TOP PRIORITY for the first several months of your new keto lifestyle.

BREATH

Special breathalyzers can detect acetone molecules in the air flowing through them. The presence of acetone in the air leaving your lungs means you have extra ketones. When acetone is in your breath you are in ketosis. This innovative tool has many advantages and will likely continue to grow in popularity.

BLOOD

Measuring your blood ketones is the best way to know if you are in ketosis. Unlike the extra, wasted ketones found in your urine or breath, ketones in your blood are a direct measurement of your ketone energy supply. This test measures the ketone Beta-hydroxybutyrate, abbreviated BHB.

Thankfully, you don't need to go to a lab or hospital to measure BHB. Home monitors, like those used by diabetics to measure blood sugars, are available without a prescription. Prick your finger and assess your ketone level in that blood drop. Within seconds, you have your answer. Real-time, accurate feedback. At the first mention of finger-pricking and self-testing, many patients get cold feet. Don't. The process can seem intrusive at first glance. However, my most successful patients embraced the accountability made possible by self-monitoring. Much like stepping on a scale provides feedback, so does testing your blood ketones and blood glucose.

Best Ketones for Adapting

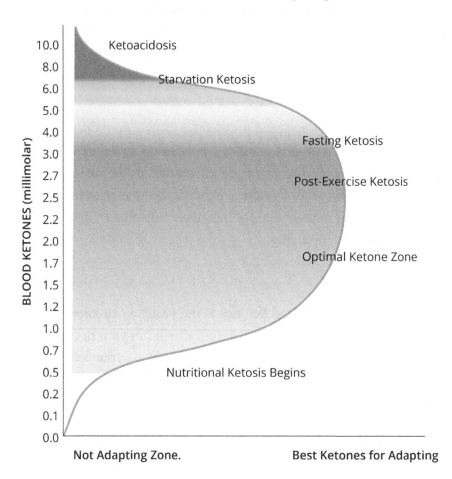

Ketone blood levels range from 0.5 to 10 millimoles per liter. Any number greater than 0.5 mmol/L translates to nutritional ketosis. Good job!

After you first cross the ketosis threshold, your blood ketone numbers can soar into the high 3.0-6.0 mmol/L range. As your cells remember how to process a 'new' fuel type, your BHB numbers settle into the 0.5-1.5 mmol/L range.

Blood ketone levels have different ranges for different goals. Urine ketone sticks turn positive when blood ketones are 0.5 mmol/L or higher. My recommendations are:

Weight-loss: above 0.5 mmol/L

Improved athletic performance: above 0.5 mmol/L

Improved mental performance: 1.0-3 mmol/L

Therapeutic (e.g., to help with specific medical problems): 2-6 mmol/L

BLOOD KETONE TESTING

PRO	CON
Most precise measurement. Direct measurement of the ketones, not a by product of the fuel.	Ketone blood test strips are expensive ranging $4-$10 PER test strip.
Trustworthy results.	Limited availability. Blood ketone testing strips found through internet. Not in local stores.
Researchers use this form of ketone measurement for data. Most scientific.	Requires a finger prick.

Personally, I began blood testing after six months. I needed an accurate and real-time method that kept me accountable.

To help you decide which testing method to go with, here are the pros and cons of each of the three methods.

URINE KETONE TESTING

PROS	CONS
Least expensive method	Urine strips measure ketones passed out as waste instead of the actual ketone fuel available for your cells.
Painless	Urine strips are not always accurate. If the strips are exposed to air for too long, they go bad. Buy them in small quantities and be sure to tightly close the bottle.
Delivers results in seconds.	Can't always trust the negative results. [Possible false negative results.] After keto adaptation, your system uses ketones more efficiently. You may use ketones as fuel, but not waste any extras into your urine. This would show no ketones in your urine, but your body continues to produce and use ketones.
Place 3-4 strips in your pocket. When using the bathroom throughout the day, check your ketones.	Faulty results. As urine collects in your bladder, ketones spilled into the bladder during that time. Those ketones turn the test positive. The positive test reports you made ketones during the time you made the urine. It does not tell you when your body was in ketosis. It only shows you that you made ketones since the last time you voided.

You should ALWAYS be able to turn the urine strip slightly pink. Urine ketone strips are great for proving you are in ketosis. Don't heavily rely on urine ketone strips to tell you HOW MUCH ketones you are making. Once keto adapted, you can't trust the amount measured by the urine strips, only whether you are in ketosis or not.
Personally, the level of ketones is a distraction for most of my patients. Stay focused on making ketones. That's it.

BREATH KETONE TESTING

PRO	CON
Very easy to perform.	Limited availability. Sold only online.
Accuracy is close to the blood test version but not quite as accurate.	Not everyone can blow into a meter for 10-30 sec straight.
Breathalyzer costs are upfront. After purchase, you can test as many times as you want without spending another dime.	Measures wasted ketone fuel instead of useable ketones.
Completely painless.	

Chapter 15

Grandma Rose: ... AND THEN WE FAILED

In the spirit of living the rest of her life to the fullest, Grandma Rose planned to check a few things off of her bucket list. Seeing a live Broadway show topped her list. Walking in New York City was off the table until she fixed the crippling bunion on her right foot. She took my repeated warnings of surgery seriously and had avoided going under the knife for all of her adult life. For ten years, her bunion evolved into a massive crisscrossing tangle of toes. Before her big trip, she elected to surgically correct that deformed mess.

There's nothing like a surgery complication to get my attention. When the surgeon walked out after three hours in the operating room for a procedure that should have taken him 15 minutes, I knew.

"Have you ever put a screw into soft, wet particle board?" That's how the surgeon described Grandma Rose's bones in her foot. His attempt to anchor the correction of her bunion was derailed by her 'mushy' bones.

What should have been a common and simple procedure had now turned into six weeks of no weight-bearing, using crutches, and a shoddy immune system.

Surgery at age 72 always draws concerns about an infection. Grandma Rose's toe supplied a dreamland for bugs looking for an easy meal and refuge. Because the screws could not hold her foot together, the surgeon slid several wires through her mushy bones. These wires went through her foot and anchored the toes to the cage surrounding her foot.

In theory, the cage formed the immovable structure that held the wires in place until her bones started to weave back together. The flaw in this theory screamed at all of us the first time Grandma Rose bumped her cage. The pain vibrated down the wires rattling the inside tunnels of her toe bones. In case that wasn't enough, these wires also provided a direct pathway for infections.

Every surgery leaves a vulnerable entrance for infections to enter. The scalpel sliced through your best defense against invasion: your skin. A healthy young person's body would seal that opening within a few days. Age slowed down that sealing process for Grandma Rose. So did her rotten CLL immune system. So did the swelling.

Six weeks. No bumping the foot. No bearing any weight on her foot. No exposure to infections while living on the farm. Oh, and let us not forget: don't allow her CLL to get worse.

Full-court ketosis press, here we come again.

"Doc, what would you do?"

As that question circled inside my mind, I scolded myself for allowing her to have the surgery. Those mangled toes would not have killed her. But this mess might. As I considered all of her situations, she faced an uncomfortably high chance of amputation. Her risks for these extreme outcomes decreased if she did not get an infection, if the swelling reversed and if her bones healed without complications. These seemed to be too much to ask for in her situation.

My Best Answer: Keto eating with half of a can of sardines every day for six weeks.

Yep. We added sardines to Grandma Rose's daily foods. For real. Not only was this a very high source of absorbable calcium to help those mushy bones, but sardines in oil were keto. Like a trooper, Grandma Rose told herself she would learn to like sardines. With the return of these complications, Dad was willing to get back on the keto bandwagon again. He gladly ate the other half of her sardines.

The weeks that followed proved to be the most teachable part of Grandma Rose's journey. The landmines that riddled her path remained hidden because they never happened. There is no way she should have done as well as she did after this debacle. The level of danger in her situation pointed to disaster no matter how I approached it. With two decades of practicing the ability to predict medical disasters, this case was a slam dunk. At 72 years old, Grandma Rose had a toe filled with crumbled, mushy bones, an open wound with wires guiding infection into one of the most sterile parts of the human body and an immune system functioning so poorly, she could not be trusted to defend herself against the wimpiest of invaders. Grandma Rose had a 100% chance of a poor outcome.

But the transformation happening at a cellular level resulted in repeated blessings. There was something much more profound happening deep inside her body since she started producing ketones. She healed completely, flawlessly and without one single complication. Impossible.

Three months after the mushy toe surgery, just before Christmas, Grandma Rose checked off that Broadway Show from her bucket list. With the help of her ketones and sardines, her toe had mended perfectly.

Her CLL numbers continued to slowly rise.

Her renewed discipline to pee ketones started to produce other benefits that were far less important to us, but noticeable.

Grandma Rose had lost 25 pounds since going keto. It had been nearly seven months since the start of her keto transition. She lost weight slowly, but effortlessly. Despite the growth of her decaying immune cells, her skin glowed with the radiance that matched the image I saw in her wedding photo. Her focus and memory were as sharp as before she developed cancer. Lock a 72-year-old woman up in a recliner for six weeks with no weight-bearing while isolated inside a rural farmhouse and even Mary Poppins risked depression.

But she did well. Very well. Her mind, energy, and mood amazed me.

All these little changes showed in Grandma Rose. She looked and felt and behaved like the woman I remember as a teenager. She was radiant.

Chapter 16

Lessons from Dr. Bosworth:
YOUR KETO TRANSITION ROADMAP

If Ketosis or Ketogenic Diets are so AWESOME, why isn't everyone on this type of diet?

ANSWER: The transition from glucose to fat can be rough for many.

Compare these two charts.

Both charts plot out several of the most common diets and compare them to one another. The first chart compares the percentage of carbohydrates in each diet versus the percentage of protein. The second one plots the percentage of fats along the bottom with the carbohydrate percentage on the left.

Notice the Standard American Diet (SAD) in both charts. On the SAD, carbohydrates make up 60% of your fuel. This diet packs 300 grams of sugar-based fuel into your body. Every single cell in your body is fueled by glucose when you eat this way. From your brain to your skin, your system uses sugar for energy. That's a lot of burning pine needles. Switch from sugar to fat, and that shift in power-source can make a mighty crabby person.

The Paleo diet has been used by many of my patients. This diet generally limits the carbohydrates to under 30% of the total food. Patients benefit from this lower amount of carbohydrates, but never fully arrive at the improved chemistry environment found with ketosis. If the dieter is lean, they often have lots of praise to say about the paleo diet. However, if they are more than a few pounds overweight, their insulin system over-shoots producing way more insulin than needed. They have been squirting insulin at extra carbs for years. Their insulin levels are high enough to lock down the fat inside that layer of pudginess. Those fat cells are stuffed full and there to stay until the insulin sinks low enough. That continuously elevated insulin leaves them with cravings and a constant cycle of insulin chasing carbs.

When you dramatically reduce your carbohydrate count, your body experiences a hormonal shift-with insulin leading the way. The cycle stops with the near-removal of carbohydrates.

Some patients eat as much as 300 or 400 grams of carbohydrates in a day when they first come to my clinic. Twenty carbs per day is a massive drop for most Americans. When you stop eating carbohydrates, keto transition begins.

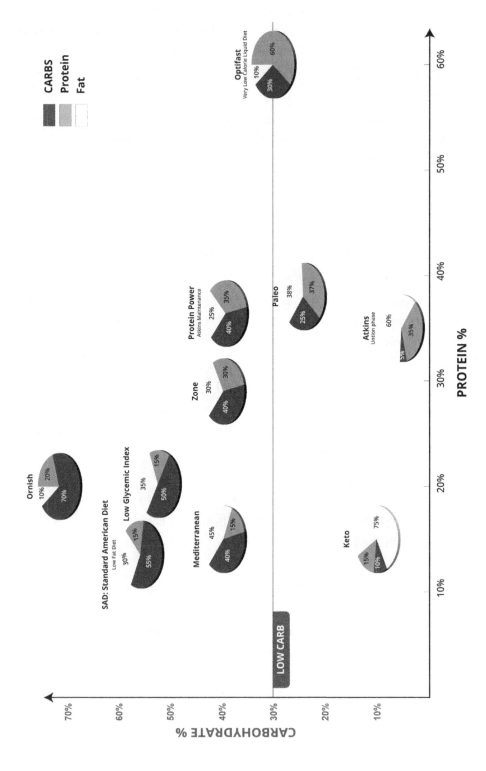

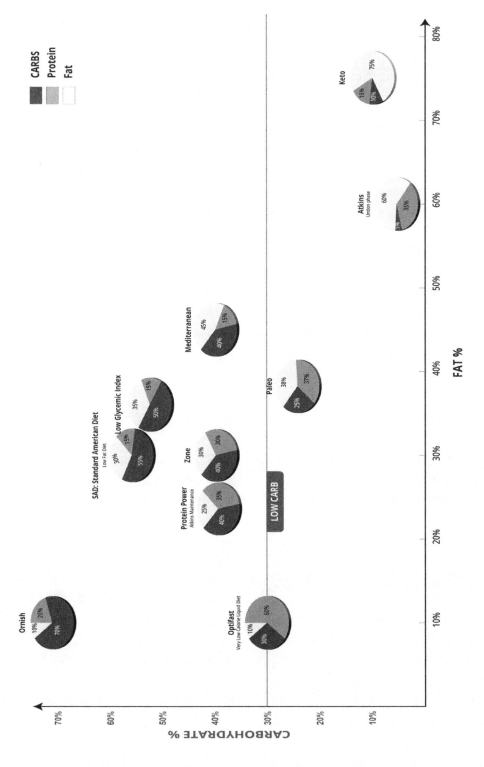

HOW TO TRANSITION TO A KETO-FUELED SYSTEM

Making the switch involves the phases described below. Each phase involves marked changes in your blood chemistry and occurs at different times.

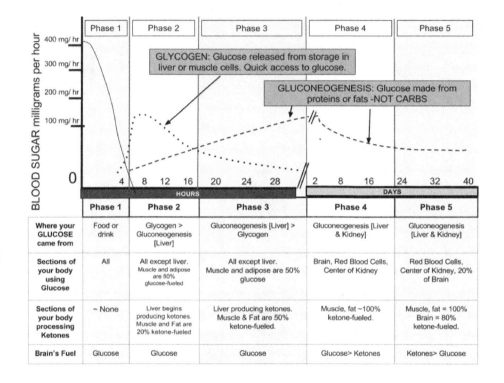

	Phase 1	Phase 2	Phase 3	Phase 4	Phase 5
Where your GLUCOSE came from	Food or drink	Glycogen > Gluconeogenesis [Liver]	Gluconeogenesis [Liver] > Glycogen	Gluconeogenesis [Liver & Kidney]	Gluconeogenesis [Liver & Kidney]
Sections of your body using Glucose	All	All except liver. Muscle and adipose are 80% glucose-fueled	All except liver. Muscle and adipose are 50% glucose	Brain, Red Blood Cells, Center of Kidney	Red Blood Cells, Center of Kidney, 20% of Brain
Sections of your body processing Ketones	~ None	Liver begins producing ketones. Muscle and Fat are 20% ketone-fueled	Liver producing ketones. Muscle & Fat are 50% ketone-fueled.	Muscle, fat ~100% ketone-fueled.	Muscle, fat = 100% Brain = 80% ketone-fueled.
Brain's Fuel	Glucose	Glucose	Glucose	Glucose> Ketones	Ketones> Glucose

PHASE 1 USE SUGAR IN BLOOD

BURN THROUGH THE SUGAR IN YOUR BLOOD
TIME REQUIRED: 4 HOURS
STATUS: Your fuel is 100% glucose. It comes from the carbs you just ate or drank. NOT ONE section of your body runs off ketones.
BRAIN: Powered only by glucose.

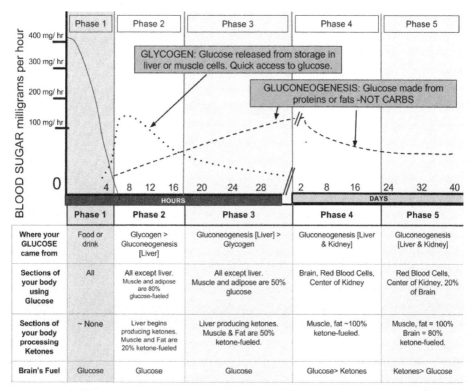

	Phase 1	Phase 2	Phase 3	Phase 4	Phase 5
Where your GLUCOSE came from	Food or drink	Glycogen > Gluconeogenesis [Liver]	Gluconeogenesis [Liver] > Glycogen	Gluconeogenesis [Liver & Kidney]	Gluconeogenesis [Liver & Kidney]
Sections of your body using Glucose	All	All except liver. Muscle and adipose are 80% glucose-fueled	All except liver. Muscle and adipose are 50% glucose	Brain, Red Blood Cells, Center of Kidney	Red Blood Cells, Center of Kidney, 20% of Brain
Sections of your body processing Ketones	~ None	Liver begins producing ketones. Muscle and Fat are 20% ketone-fueled	Liver producing ketones. Muscle & Fat are 50% ketone-fueled.	Muscle, fat ~100% ketone-fueled.	Muscle, fat = 100% Brain = 80% ketone-fueled.
Brain's Fuel	Glucose	Glucose	Glucose	Glucose> Ketones	Ketones> Glucose

Entering phase 1 is the easiest part of this process. You simply use up the sugar that's currently in your bloodstream. Every time you eat more than a spoonful of sugar or a handful of carbs you reset your system back to the beginning of Phase 1.

Phase 1 begins by processing the glucose that's already in your blood. This glucose came from the food you ate over the last 4 hours.

Phase 1 is short. It ends after 4 hours, unless you reset things by eating more carbs. Then it starts over. Don't do that.

Go to bed two hours after your last carbohydrate. Before you wake up, you are through Phase 1.

Congratulations.

PHASE 2 BURN SUGAR STORED IN LIVER

YOUR LIVER MAKES GLUCOSE BY EMPTYING ITS STORED SUGAR
TIME: 12+ HOURS
STATUS: Your fuel is still 100% glucose, but now your carb fuel is coming from your stored sugar called glycogen.
BRAIN: Powered only by glucose.

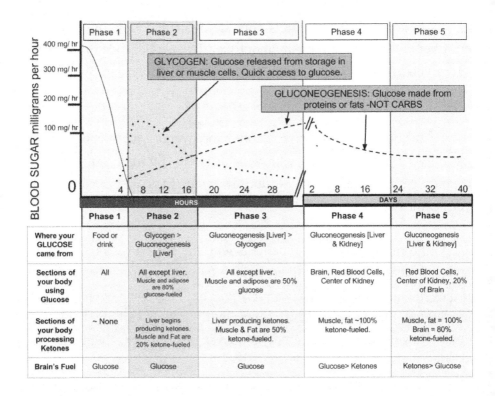

Where your GLUCOSE came from	Phase 1	Phase 2	Phase 3	Phase 4	Phase 5
Where your GLUCOSE came from	Food or drink	Glycogen > Gluconeogenesis [Liver]	Gluconeogenesis [Liver] > Glycogen	Gluconeogenesis [Liver & Kidney]	Gluconeogenesis [Liver & Kidney]
Sections of your body using Glucose	All	All except liver. Muscle and adipose are 80% glucose-fueled	All except liver. Muscle and adipose are 50% glucose	Brain, Red Blood Cells, Center of Kidney	Red Blood Cells, Center of Kidney, 20% of Brain
Sections of your body processing Ketones	~ None	Liver begins producing ketones. Muscle and Fat are 20% ketone-fueled	Liver producing ketones. Muscle & Fat are 50% ketone-fueled.	Muscle, fat ~100% ketone-fueled.	Muscle, fat = 100% Brain = 80% ketone-fueled.
Brain's Fuel	Glucose	Glucose	Glucose	Glucose> Ketones	Ketones> Glucose

You burned up those circulating sugars in your bloodstream. With no more food coming into the body through your mouth, your system will use your stored sugar. This stored sugar is called glycogen, and you keep it in your liver cells. Phase 2 fuels your body using this stored energy.

How long will your storage of glycogen last? Good question.

The answer depends on a couple of things: the size of your liver and the level of energy usage in Phase 2. Sleeping during this phase takes less fuel than running for 45 minutes. Fighting cancer or infection requires more fuel than living without those issues. Mending a broken bone or repairing from surgery requires more energy than sitting at your desk writing a book.

In addition, how large is your storage tank? How big is your liver? I bet you've never thought about that. Its size depends on how much stress you've put on it in recent years. Your liver constantly grows new cells to meet your body's needs.

If you drink excessive alcohol for twenty years, you will make more liver cells to keep up with your drinking. Similarly, if you eat lots of extra carbohydrates for two decades, your liver will expand to store your extra sugar.

From my experience, patients with the largest livers are not alcoholics. Instead, the biggest livers belong to my patients addicted to carbs. If they are not already diabetics, they will be. They have overstuffed their livers with the age-old habit of constantly eating carbohydrates. They don't allow enough time to empty stored sugars before eating more.

Long before diabetics are diagnosed, their livers strain from the pressure of the carbs they eat. They make more and more liver cells to keep up with the carbohydrate onslaught. If they cannot make extra liver cells as fast as they overeat, sugar remains in their bloodstream longer than normal. Insulin works overtime whipping the glucose into the mitochondria's furnaces or into storage. The danger signal of insulin rings constantly. They keep eating and therefore more sugars enter the bloodstream before the abundant pine needle-like fuel gets burned or stored. The screaming alarm signal of insulin becomes a constant noise. This hormone's danger signal becomes less and less effective as blood sugars steadily rise.

Diabetes is defined as a state of constantly elevated blood sugars. Diabetics never empty their storage. Their liver cells are stuffed with glycogen. Their cells have no more room. In an attempt to store their extra sugar, they grow more liver cells.

Did you empty your liver last night? Let's check. After 12 hours with only water, prick your finger and check your fasting blood sugar.

Don't roll your eyes. You must know someone who has diabetes and checks their blood sugar. Borrow their glucose monitor for one day. No, they won't die if they don't check for a day.

If you burned through all your glycogen and emptied your storage-emptied your liver- your fasting sugars will fall between 55-80 mg/dL. That's a surefire sign you have a normal sized liver. If your liver has been stretched and stuffed with too many extra carbs in recent years, you won't burn through all the storage in 12 hours. It might take you 20 hours to burn all those pine needles. Some severely overweight patients take a week. If your blood sugar is greater than 120 mg/dL at 12 hours of fasting, you have DIABETES. No joke! That's the rule of how to diagnose a diabetic.

Ideally, your liver should deplete all stored sugar before you eat another bite of food, especially foods filled with carbs. By the end of Phase 2, your body has burned all of your fast-burning fuel.

PHASE 3 YOUR LIVER STARTS MAKING KETONES

TIME: 24 HOURS
STATUS: Your fuel is still mostly glucose, but your liver begins making ketones. Only a couple of sections use ketones as fuel.
BRAIN: Still powered only by glucose.

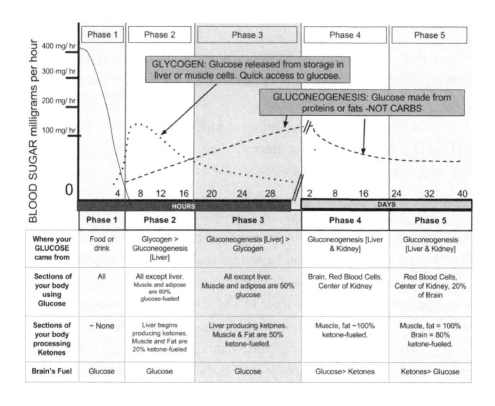

	Phase 1	Phase 2	Phase 3	Phase 4	Phase 5
Where your GLUCOSE came from	Food or drink	Glycogen > Gluconeogenesis [Liver]	Gluconeogenesis [Liver] > Glycogen	Gluconeogenesis [Liver & Kidney]	Gluconeogenesis [Liver & Kidney]
Sections of your body using Glucose	All	All except liver. Muscle and adipose are 80% glucose-fueled	All except liver. Muscle and adipose are 50% glucose	Brain, Red Blood Cells, Center of Kidney	Red Blood Cells, Center of Kidney, 20% of Brain
Sections of your body processing Ketones	~ None	Liver begins producing ketones. Muscle and Fat are 20% ketone-fueled	Liver producing ketones. Muscle & Fat are 50% ketone-fueled.	Muscle, fat ~100% ketone-fueled.	Muscle, fat = 100% ketone-fueled. Brain = 80% ketone-fueled.
Brain's Fuel	Glucose	Glucose	Glucose	Glucose> Ketones	Ketones> Glucose

You will know the exact point when you complete Phase 2 and enter Phase 3. How? You start peeing ketones! Transitioning from Phase 2 to 3 happens at different times for different people because of the liver's variables described above.

Here are some common statements from patients that tip me off to the possibility that they may have an overstuffed liver:

'Doctor, I have tried every diet. None of them worked.'

'Doctor, I am a dude, and I look pregnant. Can you fix this?'

'Doc, I had a gastric bypass and lost a bunch of weight... but I gained most of it back.'

These patients have a biochemistry crisis hidden inside their livers. They have had gastric bypass, gastric banding or their jaws stapled shut and still were not able to achieve lasting weight loss. They are patients who have used speed pills and antidepressants, participated in group therapy, undergone hypnosis, and injected hormones to lose weight. All share the same result: zero to minimal weight loss. Alternatively, those that lost some weight gained it all back sooner or later. They were all fighting the hidden monster of the chemistry that blocks against weight loss. The name of that enemy: insulin. The medical term for these patients is *insulin resistance* but I tell them that they have stubborn livers.

If you pee ketones by the end of the second day of cutting out carbs, do a little dance. You are not likely to be the owner of a stubborn liver. Keep track of how long it takes you to get to Phase 3. This time-to-first-urine-ketone predicts the size of your liver. Much like your fasting blood glucose results, this information tells you and your medical team what has been happening under the surface.

What is the key? Reduce your daily carbs to 20 grams or less. This shocks your sugar-dependent system. In Phase 1, every cell in your body fueled their furnaces with glucose; specifically, your brain is 100% dependent on sugar.

In Phase 3, certain parts of your body switch to using ketones for fuel. The first tissues to adapt are your fat cells and your muscles.

Other sections of your body are more protective of which fuel they use. Those tissues wait to see if this ketone fuel will be available only temporarily or long term.

Here's a cell ranking from most to least adaptable to use ketones: fat cells, muscles, skin, internal organs (heart, lungs and kidneys) and brain.

The brain is the most resistant to fuel transition and is the absolute last to convert to fat-based energy. When the brain finally switches over though--it feels good. SO GOOD!

Here is the play by play transition that I recommend for you. Just follow these steps.

Eat your final carb-based-meal and a couple of hours later go to bed.

When you awake, you are nearly 10 hours into your transition.

Within the next 12 hours, your liver will empty your stored sugar.

Throughout the day, use MCT C8:C10 oil or heavy whipping cream in your coffee. Drink water. Eat all the eggs you want. Cook them in butter.

Eat a couple of sausage patties or bacon for lunch. For work, take along some high fat cheese and slices of pepperoni in case you feel like eating in between meals.

That evening, go out to eat and order Buffalo Wings dipped in Blue Cheese dressing. Be sure to order the wings in buffalo sauce and not honey mustard or barbecue sauce. Those have carbs in them. You want the buffalo sauce. Eat wings until you are full. No beer. No soft drinks.

No breading on your Buffalo Wings. Keep the skin on. Double dip them in blue cheese dressing. Add only water for a drink.

By 8 o'clock that night, your liver should be completely cleared of glycogen. It should be completely cleared of stored sugar. Your early adapting organs will gradually begin to switch their fuel source to ketones.

Go straight to bed. Forget about getting a carb-rich snack like you're used to. If you followed my instructions, your cupboards should be emptied of all those temptations anyway.

Just go straight to bed.

You've made it 24 hours since your last helping of carbohydrates. These next 12 hours are best dealt with by sleeping and staying SOBER: Don't drink booze. Touch any alcohol and you can kiss ketosis goodbye. JUST GO TO BED!

I have had some patients in bed by 8:00 PM because they did not know how else to get off their normal routine. I don't care how you do it, just get to the next morning.

Wake up the next morning. It's been 36 hours since your last high dose of carbohydrates. This puts you almost always into Phase 3. Check your ketone strips. Even a slightly pink color on the strip is a win.

Stubborn livers beware! If your liver is overworked, stretched out or engorged with stored sugar, you might not be there yet. If you've been a really big carb junkie, overweight for many years, or a full blown diabetic, you might have another day ahead before your ketone test turns positive.

<u>Make this your morning ritual</u>: Check your ketone urine strip.

Put 4 more strips in your pocket. These break down when exposed to air for too long. You have only that day to use the strips in your pocket.   Otherwise, throw them away. Each time you pee, check your urine for ketones.

Use those ketone strips to see exactly which phase you are in. Are you in Phase 2 or have you arrived at Phase 3? The answer is hidden unless you look.

Before I insisted that patients check their ketones, several patients who needed this lifestyle the most gave up. I lost them to frustration. This sets in when you don't know what is going on inside your system. Changing eating patterns shocks the daily routine of most patients. They are delighted when the results hit them - mentally and physically. But if the results never come, frustration leads to failure. They ask for my help, and I need reliable information in order to help them. Keep track of how long it takes your liver to empty. Check your urine ketones.

My experience with peeing my first ketone involved a full month of frustration. I was insulin resistant and then I ate too much protein. I realized I had one of those stubborn livers. I was also unaware of the carbohydrates hidden in gum, toothpaste, cough drops and sauces. I didn't know the mayonnaise I was using had carbs in it. I also ate soups made with flour. I would be doing well and then BAM-no more ketones.

Had I not been looking at that urine ketone strip the first month, I would have certainly given up. The mistakes I was making would have been unknown without that feedback.

CHECK YOUR URINE KETONES SEVERAL TIMES A DAY FOR THE FIRST FEW WEEKS.

PHASE 4 TRANSITIONING

TIME: 2 WEEKS
STATUS: Your fuel is now a blend of ketones and glucose. Gradually more sections use ketones as fuel.
BRAIN: Powered mostly by glucose, but a few cells use ketones.

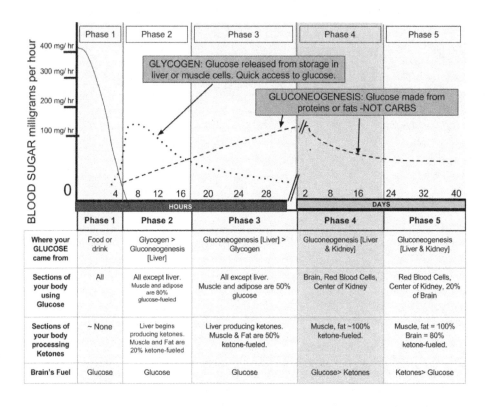

	Phase 1	Phase 2	Phase 3	Phase 4	Phase 5
Where your GLUCOSE came from	Food or drink	Glycogen > Gluconeogenesis [Liver]	Gluconeogenesis [Liver] > Glycogen	Gluconeogenesis [Liver & Kidney]	Gluconeogenesis [Liver & Kidney]
Sections of your body using Glucose	All	All except liver. Muscle and adipose are 80% glucose-fueled	All except liver. Muscle and adipose are 50% glucose	Brain, Red Blood Cells, Center of Kidney	Red Blood Cells, Center of Kidney, 20% of Brain
Sections of your body processing Ketones	~ None	Liver begins producing ketones. Muscle and Fat are 20% ketone-fueled	Liver producing ketones. Muscle & Fat are 50% ketone-fueled.	Muscle, fat ~100% ketone-fueled.	Muscle, fat = 100% Brain = 80% ketone-fueled.
Brain's Fuel	Glucose	Glucose	Glucose	Glucose> Ketones	Ketones> Glucose

This phase of this process focuses on converting stubborn parts of your body to burn fat for fuel. Your ketone resistant cells begin transitioning. By Phase 4 your liver is really good at making ketones. Your blood abounds with these compounds. Slowly the rusty, unused cell parts that make and burn ketones come to life. If we checked your blood we would find a hearty amount of ketones ranging from 2-3 mMol/dl.

As the liver pumps out a steady stream of this fuel, the rest of your body is still getting used to processing it. Over the two weeks of Phase 4, your ketone efficiency catches up with your liver's abundant production. By the end of this phase, your blood ketones will settle into the 0.5-1.5 mMol/dl range.

Now might be a good time to remind you why in the world those ketones are in your urine. Weren't you supposed to make ketones to fuel your body? Why are they in your urine? Why didn't we keep them all in the blood circulating around?

When you are in Phase 4, the mismatch between how well your liver makes ketones and how efficiently the rest of your body uses them leaves you with too many. Your kidney closely watches your body's chemistry. If there are too many ketones around, the kidney passes them into the urine. The kidneys and your lungs act as an overflow valve for the extra.

Before you get disappointed about wasting those valuable ketones, keep in mind, they used to be fat calories. You are literally peeing out extra calories! How fun of a weight loss plan is THAT? Right on!

By the end of Phase 4, nearly every cell has processed its own ketone. They might not yet use this fuel steadily, but all of them activated their ketone burning furnaces. Even your most resistant organs have a few cells running on this fuel.

If you kept those carbs less than 20 grams per day, your storage tank is sure to be empty. Your body makes glucose less and less as more cells use ketones instead.

Wait a minute. If you're not eating carbs and you burned through all the ones you had in storage, where is all this glucose coming from?

ANSWER: It is coming from your fat too. Your fat chains, called fatty acids, travel in groups of three chains. These 3 chains are held together by a little glucose-based molecule. Your liver clips off the fat to turn into ketones. A very small amount of glucose is left over. This tiny source of glucose is saved for your stubborn organs that have a difficult time switching over to pure ketones.

PHASE 5 KETO-ADAPTED

TIME: THE REST OF YOUR LIFE
STATUS: Your fuel is mostly ketones with a sprinkle of glucose.
BRAIN: Powered mostly by ketones, but still uses glucose.

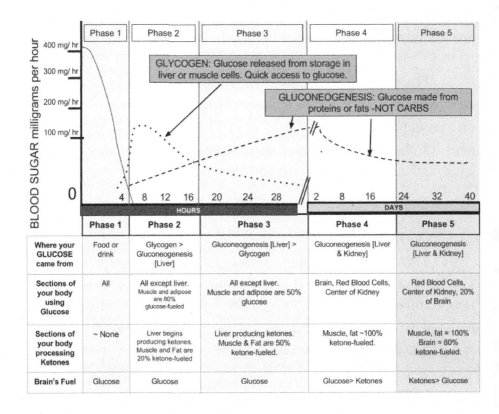

	Phase 1	Phase 2	Phase 3	Phase 4	Phase 5
Where your GLUCOSE came from	Food or drink	Glycogen > Gluconeogenesis [Liver]	Gluconeogenesis [Liver] > Glycogen	Gluconeogenesis [Liver & Kidney]	Gluconeogenesis [Liver & Kidney]
Sections of your body using Glucose	All	All except liver. Muscle and adipose are 80% glucose-fueled	All except liver. Muscle and adipose are 50% glucose	Brain, Red Blood Cells, Center of Kidney	Red Blood Cells, Center of Kidney, 20% of Brain
Sections of your body processing Ketones	~ None	Liver begins producing ketones. Muscle and Fat are 20% ketone-fueled	Liver producing ketones. Muscle & Fat are 50% ketone-fueled.	Muscle, fat ~100% ketone-fueled.	Muscle, fat = 100% Brain = 80% ketone-fueled.
Brain's Fuel	Glucose	Glucose	Glucose	Glucose> Ketones	Ketones> Glucose

Phase 5 is when your body becomes the well-oiled machine it was designed to be. Each mitochondria able to use ketones now efficiently handles this fuel type. Thanks to the steady, constant supply of ketones your cells efficiency to process them increased. They are produced and burned at almost equal rates. Because your production and usage are better matched, ketones no longer circulate as long. Phase 5 is marked by a significant drop in your blood ketones. Subsequently, the amount spilling into your urine drops, too.

In a rare moment, your ketone production and usage match perfectly, leaving no extras in your urine. This can be tricky if you are only checking urine ketones. Did your ketones stop showing up in your urine because you ate a bunch of carbs? Drank booze? Maybe the bottle of strips was left open and went bad? Or did your urine ketones stop appearing because your system had a perfect match? Rest assured, the first three options are much more likely.

Phase 5 is the holy grail. Once your brain reaches this state, you will better appreciate all the hype surrounding a ketosis lifestyle. It borders on euphoric. When patients enter Phase 5, their depression symptoms lift, their focus improves, their attention lasts longer, their sleep is more restful, and their energy is contagious.

How do you get to Phase 5?

There is a fast way and a slower way. The fast way is a strict fast. That is not a play on words. I am referring to the absence of food. A strict fast is a time of no calories. Only water, tea, or coffee. That's all. Strictly limit yourself to only those items and you will be at Phase 5 in about 30 or 40 days. That's a tough sell.

I DO NOT recommend this option. Especially if you are eating a high-carbohydrate diet right now. High carbohydrate means eating over 60 carb grams per day. There are just too many shifts that have to happen in your system. It's too unsettling, too uncomfortable, and in many of my chronically ill patients, it is dangerous.

Instead, transition into Phase 5 using a high fat diet. Patients transition to a high-fat diet and pee ketones for several weeks. This allows time to adjust. It also provides time to see how much social pressure is placed on eating carbohydrates and low-fat foods.

KETOADAPTATION
METABOLIC BENEFITS

WHEN: 2-4 WEEKS AFTER STEADY KETONE PRODUCTION	INCREASE NUMBER OF FUNCTIONING MITOCHONDRIA [All mitochondria are adding energy to the system]
WHAT: A SHIFT IN BODY'S METABOLISM WHERE THE BODY PREFERS KETONES AS FUEL	WEIGHT LOSS WITH LEANER BODY COMPOSITION [Lose fat, not muscle]
GLYCOGEN HORMONE = LOWERED [Glycogen = glucose stored in muscles and liver]	INCREASE INSULIN SENSITIVITY [Small amounts of insulin needed for body to respond]
DECREASED FATIGUE	FASTER REPAIR OF THE BODY
ENHANCE BRAIN ENERGY	IMPROVE EFFICIENCY OF OXYGEN DELIVERY TO MUSCLE CELLS
REDUCE FREE RADICALS	FASTER RECOVERY TIME
BOOST BASELINE ENERGY [Due to steady ketone supply feeding mitochondria]	

*Volek et al
Strength & condition J. 32:42-47, 2010*

Screw-ups happen often when first eating high-fat low-carb. They drink alcohol. They eat too much protein. They get stingy on their fat consumption. They mindlessly binge on ice cream after a stressful day. Or someone near them celebrates an occasion with sugary treats, and the temptation becomes too great at the moment. The bottom line? Changing habits is hard.

The idea that a smoker wakes up one day and stops smoking for the rest of his life is a fantasy. That person who 'suddenly' quits smoking had months, maybe even years, of thoughts and false starts about quitting before they actually stopped. Their environment played a big role in their success. If their world tempted them with cigarettes at every turn, their chances of achieving a smoke-free life one year later are very unlikely. People in keto transition need support. Without it, temptations win out.

That is my goal: a healthy life. Not a sprint to ketone positive urine tests. The key to sustainability is the LONG GAME.

Ultimately, it doesn't matter whether you get to Phase 5 in 6 weeks or 6 months. Boost your chances of lifelong success by keeping your priorities straight. Remember why you decided to go keto in the first place. Write it down. Say it out loud.

My personal reason for going keto: Brain fuel, brain fuel, brain fuel.

Chapter 17
Grandma Rose: BOWEL TROUBLE

Ten years ago on New Year's Eve, Grandma Rose's holiday cocktail dripped into her veins. She rested in darkness as intravenous lines filled her with pain meds, antibiotics, and saline. The pathology lab doctor entered the back stairwell. His heavy feet echoed each step as he went through the floors from the basement to third. In the isolation of his climb, he rehearsed what he would say to Grandma Rose. He entered her room late that night with news that changed her life.

Severe abdominal pain drove her into the emergency room. A CT scan showed pockets of infected diverticula along the last section of her colon. The pathologist found her deformed white blood cells and understood why her body struggled to defend against the infection. He delivered the news she had cancer just before the calendar year turned.

Each New Year's celebration since, we toasted to another year. Grandma Rose rang in the New Year with abundant gratitude.

This year's chapter of her CLL story started with the return to the beginning: a flare in those pockets lining her colon.

Her cancer had grown quite a bit in the past year. Our secret cancer-starving keto plan swatted away chemo at least twice in 12 months, but we knew it wouldn't be long before another round was needed. Her bone marrow told the clearest story of what was happening.

Inside her bone marrow, she grew some red blood cells (RBC), some white blood cells (WBC), and some platelets. The cancerous white blood cells had grown so abundant that very little space remained for forming RBC or platelets.

When a high WBC count comes back on most patient's lab report, we assume they are fighting off infection. However, in Grandma Rose's case, most of the infection-fighting cells didn't work. A normal WBC number is 6,000. Her WBC number soared over 150,000, and she suffered from more and more infections. More importantly, her RBCs and platelets struggled to find the real estate inside her bones to grow. Their numbers dropped to dangerously low levels.

After ten years, Grandma Rose had hundreds of diverticula in her colon. Diverticula are abnormal balloon-shaped pockets that develop in the lower parts of our colon as we age. Although colon diverticula are abnormal, this problem happens to so many people that doctors don't consider them alarming unless these get infected. Once you get a few diverticula, it's easier to develop a few more.

In January, days after celebrating a decade of no trouble, one of Grandma Rose's diverticula got infected and swelled so much it sealed off the rest of her colon. Inside that sealed pouch collected a tiny drop of poop. It may seem small and insignificant but this condition can actually be quite deadly given Grandma Rose's weakened immune system. With her overwhelming majority of deformed white cells, we prayed for the remaining few good cells to do their job.

Epic fail.

Grandma Rose's degraded immune system lost that battle. Despite months of ketones, a half-dozen pockets of diverticula evolved into just as many abscesses lining her colon.

BUGGER!!!

We were in a jam. The infection-filled-pockets lined Grandma Rose's colon. Her crippled immune system put up little resistance as these infections conquered more of her bowel. The central tunnel where her stools passed collapsed to a sliver of an opening. In addition, her cancer had consumed nearly all the space within her bones, leaving little hope that a fresh batch of hardy white cells would arrive any time soon.

We returned to the exact same hospital room in the small town she had been in ten years prior. Heavy doses of antibiotics helped a little but could not cure the problem. The swollen infections sponged up more and more space. These abscesses needed to be drained.

I fantasized of inserting a tiny hose into each carbuncle, and sucking out all the death living there. Each scan showed the evil fruits more distended and ripe. Every medical textbook gave the same advice: 'drain or die.' The idea of more surgery forced me to swallow hard. Grandma Rose arrived at the death-bound trifecta: low blood count (RBC) combined with a weakened immune system (WBC) and a dwindling platelet count.

This puzzle had no answer that included Grandma Rose surviving. Surgery would kill her from the blood loss or the ensuing infection. Waiting was also a non-starter because the gestating infections would consume her blood and body in the short days ahead.

We needed a miracle.

Her doctors added blood transfusions, dripped in antibiotics, quieted her pain with morphine and kept her frail body well-hydrated.

Problem: Her bowels were now swollen shut. How do you stop guts from pooping?

Any food that passed the section where her poison cocoons lay waiting risked triggering a toxic explosion into her bloodstream. One drop. One leak. That's all it would take.

The solution? Stop eating. Grandma Rose needed to fast.

Grandma Rose raised our family with a solid understanding of who we were and who we were not. As Midwestern farmers, we topped the nation with our strong work ethic. As the principal of our town's Sunday School, our small, rural community depended on our family to show up and participate in all church activities. Despite our faithful devotion, not once had my family fasted. We never lacked for food. Meat and potatoes. Corn and beans. Three squares a day. Everyone in our family had the waistlines to prove it. Our loyalty to eating at set times matched our loyalty to God.

Grandma Rose's life depended upon stopping her bowel movements. Instantly, we became a family that fasted.

NPO-*nil per os*-nothing per mouth. That was Grandma Rose's new label.

Nurses called her "The NPO patient at the end of the hall." Signs reminded everyone from the hospital's CEO to the janitor not to feed or water her. She traded anything entering her mouth for that salted IV fluid slowly dripping into her veins.

To show my support, I agreed to fast with her. Without the luxury of Grandma Rose's expertly calculated electrolytes, I added several salt crystals to my pocket each morning. My antidote to waves of hunger during a fast was quick access to Himalayan Salt Crystals. Placed on the tip of my tongue, these stopped hunger pangs like a charm.

The first 48 hours were much harder for me than for Grandma Rose. Thanks to the zombie-like state of mind her pain meds produced, she doesn't remember anything about this fasting stage.

Six months of practicing ketosis prepared her body. Her cells were ready for ketone fuel. Her strict abstinence from eating calories promptly flipped her system into using her stored fat. Designed for exactly this situation, Grandma Rose's system went from using glucose, protein and fat entering into her body through her mouth, to strictly using the fat-fuel stored inside her fat cells.

Anyone of us would make this transition if we were forced to stop eating. However, because every cell in her body had been exposed to ketones for the better part of six months, Grandma Rose switched to a solid energy state producing ketones with little to no trouble. She suffered none of the crabby 'hangry' (hunger mixed with anger) symptoms often linked to this switch. When all food stopped entering her mouth, she reached for those calories squirreled inside her fat cells.

By seventy-two hours, she was doing great without any hunger pangs.

Near the eighty-sixth hour of her fast, God delivered the miracle we had prayed for.

The abscesses stewing in the depths of her pelvis combined their goo and started to drain. A miracle!

The abscesses drained!!! This was exactly what I had prayed for.

Where, you ask? Where did these abscesses deep within her pelvis drain to? In true Grandma Rose fashion, a clever, albeit unsettling, solution appeared.

Grandma's infection re-routed to the nearest opening, her birthing canal. She now pooped out her vagina!

Can you imagine that? A pooping vagina? This is not normal. None of her medical team had even heard of such an option. Nowhere in any textbooks does this idea get talked about because it was so strange. We teased her that she had taken her MacGyver skills of repurposing items throughout her lifetime of farming, self-reliance, and resourceful-ness to a whole other level.

This pooping birth canal problem was the weirdest thing. But it worked.

That night, instead of planning her funeral, I spent six hours read-ing everything I could find about extended fasts. I'm talking about fasting for 40-50 days. As delighted as I was about her pooping vagina, the reason those abscesses formed in the first place was because there was no defense system strong enough to fight those infections. Her white blood cells were useless. She needed chemo. Her crowded bone marrow needed a reset to produce space for healthy cells to grow back in. On the other hand, a dose of chemo right now would only reignite the flames inside those abscesses. We needed to get her just well enough to endure a round of chemo. We needed those bacteria within the abscesses to die off. We prayed nothing else got infected in the meantime.

We had a complicated mess on our hands. Thankfully, that's my specialty.

Chapter 18

Lessons from Dr. Bosworth:

WHAT CAN POSSIBLY GO WRONG?

If you are peeing ketones and feeling fine, skip right over this chapter.

However, if you tried to make ketones and you never turned your strip pink, read this chapter.

If you are a worrier and you read on the Internet all the ways this 'crazy' diet supposedly messes up your body, read this chapter.

Let's do a tiny recap:

A body fueled by sugar is chronically inflamed and in crisis. It is impossible to drip in the exact amount of carb fuel needed without going over or under your requirements. More than a teaspoon of carbs pushes your body into releasing insulin. When glucose is your fuel, eating too little leads to a steady decrease in your metabolism. Conversely, extra, unused glucose, rings your 'insulin alarm' triggering a spike of this hormone and continuing the cycle of inflammation.

Fueling your body with fat means no insulin. You rid yourself from the crisis. Extra, unused ketones slip through your system and lubricate your body. A state of ketosis reverses inflammation caused by chronic high insulin levels.

As an internal medicine doctor, my job is helping with your health's 'long game.' In other words, chronic disease management. When your body swells on the inside, that inflammation causes trouble. Chronic, slow-growing inflammation creeps into more and more areas of your body.

After years of too many carbohydrates, your system gets really messy on the inside. But it is stable. Your cell walls become stiff and inflexible. The 'hoses' that carry your blood are crusty and can't be easily stretched or relaxed. Reversing this chronic problem is tricky. The day you flip your energy source from carbs to fat, your body chemistry changes. This sends your crusty, stiff-albeit stable-system into flux.

Here is a short list of what can go wrong after a long-term carb addict decides to make the switch to ketones.

KETO FLU

ONSET: Starts on day 2.
DURATION: Lasts for up to a week.

If you Google any side effects of the Keto Diet, this tops the list of search results.

This condition got its name because chronically inflamed patients experience flu-like symptoms as they transition. When you get the flu, a 'bug' sets up inside your body and messes with your system. Those invaders steal your water, drink your salts, and eat up your sugar. Your tummy aches, in part, because the bugs selected your guts as their new home. Flu symptoms include headache, feeling tired, dizziness upon standing, racing heart, nausea, loss of appetite and feeling rather irritable. When you get the flu, you get dehydrated causing all those symptoms. A body switching from sugar to fat also gets dehydrated. Dehydration causes the symptoms collectively called 'keto flu.'

What's so dehydrating about producing ketones? Ketones aren't the cause. Instead, it's the lack of all those glucose molecules circulating in your system. Glucose is a huge, monster-sized molecule that flows through your veins.

Glucose acts like a sponge and holds onto water as it percolates throughout the body. Each glucose molecule holds onto hundreds of water molecules. Excess bloodstream glucose translates to thousands-even millions-of extra water molecules.

Do the math.

Check your blood sugar. Is it above 100? For every point above 100, you added thousands of extra monster-sized glucose molecules to the 7 liters of blood you hold. Now, multiply that by the hundreds of water particles clinging to each glucose.

Twenty carbs per day leads to way less glucose in your bloodstream. Less glucose holding onto that water and your body flushes that extra fluid out. Over the course of the first week, I have had patients lose 20 pounds-that's nearly three gallons of extra water.

This is weight lost through excess water removal. Have you heard this: 'The only way you lose weight on a high-fat diet or Atkins-like diet is because you lose water weight?' That's exactly what happens.

Millions of water particles lost their chemical sponges and are gone. Dehydration is defined by the rapid loss of water. This is a great thing. All that extra water inflames or irritates your body. Removing it is the right answer.

'Flu' or dehydration symptoms appear when you are caught unprepared for ketosis' water loss.

This water loss hits your kidneys like a tidal wave. Your kidneys remove water from your blood by adding it to your urine. They 'steal' salt from your bloodstream to make this happen.

Before long, you get a headache and feel really tired. You try to stand up only to suffer sudden dizziness and a pounding heart. Oftentimes, you get crabby. Welcome to the keto flu.

The antidote is easy: eat SALT, drink water and slow down.

Let's start with salt. Yes, I mean salt. Like the white stuff in the shaker on your table. I prefer pink Himalayan salt or sea salt, but common table salt will do. Salt, like fat, is an overly demonized compound.

Fat and salt are important to the Keto diet. You need to replace the fluid that belongs in your body. Knowing that keto transition sucks salt and water into your urine should motivate you to add a bit of salt to anything you eat or drink. You get dizzy because there's not enough fluid in circulation. Replace that fluid by eating and drinking with salt. If you add plain water back to your system, you will not fix the flu-like symptoms. The water will go in and flush right back out. The salt holds the proper amount of water in your circulation and corrects the dehydration. Drink salty broth to keep the keto flu away!

The next step is to slow down.

If you are reading this and considering fueling your body with fat, GREAT. Let me help you succeed. If you are a carb addict with a daily intake of more than 300 carb gram, start slowly. Begin with no bread for the first week. Then move on to zero calories in your drinks for the second week as you prepare for 'transition day.' This gives you the space to allow a gentle shift in your body chemistry to prevent keto flu. This schedule also gives you enough time to clean out your cupboards.

WARNING: BE CAREFUL IF YOU TAKE HIGH BLOOD PRESSURE MEDICATIONS

ONSET: Day 2-3
DURATION: 1-2 Weeks

If you are on blood pressure medication and you want to get off them, this lifestyle is the answer. HOWEVER, the transition can be dangerous. Prepare yourself.

My patients taking high blood pressure meds must check their own blood pressure at home. Without all those huge glucose molecules loaded with hundreds of additional water particles, your body's circulating volume drops. Not because of blood loss; because of water lost. Lower volume means less pressure. It takes far less medication to control blood pressure when all that water is gone.

Thanks to the Keto diet, helping patients get off blood pressure medication has never been easier. You must use a home blood pressure monitor though. Check your blood pressure 2-3 times a day when transitioning. As you reduce and remove carbohydrates from your diet, your blood pressure will drop quickly. Be careful. Let your doctor help you remove those blood pressure medicines as quickly as you remove the carbohydrates. In a matter of five days, I got one patient off of five of his blood pressure meds! This, of course, all depends on how strict you are at following the less-than-20-carbs-a-day rule and how long you have been a carb addict.

BOWELS: TOO SLOW [CONSTIPATION]

ONSET: Day 3-4
DURATION: Lasts until your bowels adapt to your new diet.

Drinking salted water prevents the keto flu and also helps with changes happening in your guts. I'm referring specifically to your stool. Constipation and hard bowel movements happen naturally as part of the keto transition process. With less water, your stools become dehydrated and harder. Drinking salty water helps lessen this problem.

For the first couple of weeks, patients struggle with what to eat. My salesmanship for high-fat meat must work really well, because they do a great job of loading up on fatty, greasy meat. They produce ketones, but they also get constipated. A few minutes studying the number of carbs found in fruits and vegetables teach you that corn, cantaloupe, peas, bananas, and sweet-potatoes are all no-nos.

My new keto patients usually aren't that familiar with many keto-friendly vegetables. For example, cabbage, Brussels sprouts and fresh spinach are all great additions to a keto diet. Sadly, many look at me bewildered that people actually eat that stuff. They ate yummy fatty meats, successfully peed ketones and did a little dance. Everything's awesome until day 4 when they couldn't poop. Some patients got so constipated they gave up. Prepare for this constipation challenge.

Drink salty water.

Add cabbage early.

Ingest a spoonful of dry chia seeds with some water every 2-4 hours. These little seeds swell up into a gelatinous substance and have helped many patients transition.

If you're still having a tough time with constipation, try Milk of Magnesia. This over-the-counter medication is the perfect fit for this problem. In the first weeks of keto, one of the most common salts your body will be losing is magnesium. This magnesium-filled liquid medication helps replenish your missing magnesium while boosting your stools to soften up and move along.

BRISTOL STOOL CHART

TYPE 1		SEPARATE STIFF LUMPY BITS	SEVERE CONSTIPATION
TYPE 2		SAUSAGE-LIKE MASS WITH STUCK LUMPS	MILD CONSTIPATION
TYPE 3		SAUSAGE-SHAPED LONG MASS WITH SURFACE CRACKS	NORMAL
TYPE 4		SMOOTH SURFACED LONG TUBULAR FORM	NORMAL
TYPE 5		BLOBS OF SOFT MASS WITH DEFINED EDGES	LOW FIBER
TYPE 6		RAGGED EDGE MUSHY MASS	MILD DIARRHEA
TYPE 7		LIQUID WITH NO SOLID BITS	SEVERE DIARRHEA

BOWELS: TOO FAST [DIARRHEA]
ONSET: Day 3-4
DURATION: Depends on the cause.

Most people on a keto program experience bowel problems in the form of constipation. Sometimes, people experience the other extreme: diarrhea. This is usually due to a pre-existing problem with their system.

Over the years, the US government and corporations have spent millions of dollars researching ways to help people suffering from all sorts of bowel ailments. These range from irritable bowel to bacterial overgrowth, to leaky gut syndrome. One 1970s study treated irritable bowel syndrome with a high-fat diet.

It took six months for the study's subjects to become regular. Still, the study showed that a high-fat low-carb diet is one of the cheapest and most effective ways to regulate runny stools and other bowel problems. Unfortunately, the study was small and was not funded by a big pharmaceutical company. The study did not promote any medication. The outcomes from that old trial were so promising for this taxing problem, that it led me to change how I approached my patients with bowel problems. My experience with patients suffering from irritable bowel has taught me to stick to the plan of peeing ketones for three to four months before they turn the corner.

Did you know your small bowel or small intestines are supposed to be sterile? Sterile-as in no bacteria. Your large intestines are packed with bacteria. But your small intestines are supposed to be sterile. Anxiety, stress and chronic illness all lead to poorly functioning bowels. Your small intestines can get so messed up that the bacteria normally found at the end of your intestines, in the large colon, wiggle their way into the upper portion of your digestive tract. These bacteria in the small intestine reproduce without much resistance and grow rapidly. This is called small bowel overgrowth.

When patients have small bowel overgrowth, it is not uncommon for them to lose out on fatty vitamins normally absorbed there. Because their small bowel gurgles with abundant, unwanted bacteria, they can't absorb any fat-based nutrients. I've started patients on a ketogenic life-style not knowing that they had small bowel overgrowth. A week into the change and they are miserable with uncontrolled diarrhea. They call the clinic upset and declare, "This just is NOT the diet for me!"

After checking their lab results as well as a detailed history, it turns out they often have had loose stools after eating fat for the better part of a decade. These patients report avoiding all fat because it always gives them explosive diarrhea. Such eruptions after each greasy meal kept them malnourished from their avoidance of fat. They go on for years without understanding what was truly happening to their system. One day, they happen to have their Vitamin D checked. Their results were so low, it can only mean they have not been absorbing any fat for years. Fat absorption failure means you absorb no fat-based vitamins. Vitamin D is one of those vitamins.

I advise patients of mine who suffer diarrhea after switching to a high-fat diet not to give up. Why? They need this anti-inflammatory diet more than most of my other patients. If you suffer from loose stools or explosive diarrhea after going keto, give your body time to adjust. Don't give up! The health of your brain and bowels are depending on it. If your bowels flare up when switching to high fat, please know that it is more than just an annoyance. Something more is going on. Go see a gastro specialist. This extreme intestinal inflammation can last weeks. Years of this hidden problem led to the chronic swelling of your bowels' inner lining. It takes time to mend that chronic wound inside your guts.

If you get diarrhea within days of switching to keto, you have a problem with inflammation. Don't quit. Fix it.

To tide you over, I recommend the following:

Loperamide: This over the counter medication slows down bowel movements. Most people cannot put their life on hold to deal with intense diarrhea. It takes time to fix this problem. In the meantime, don't take all this suffering lying down. Control your symptoms. Take Loperamide. The brand name of this is Imodium®. This will settle the symptoms down while we work through the problem without hurting you.

Kombucha Tea: This ancient drink is a bubbly, fermented beverage with healthy live bacteria in it. Most of my diarrhea patients reversed their bowel problems when they repopulated their gut bacteria. Many patients spend thousands of dollars on this process. Save your money. Drink 1/4 of a cup of this tea a day until the diarrhea is resolved. Notice that I said ONE FOURTH OF A CUP. Too much of that bacteria is often not tolerated by those struggling with bowel problems.

Finally, the surefire antidote that transitions my diarrhea patients through the roughest part can be unsettling for patients to hear: intermittent fasting. Yes, I am referring to the term for NO EATING. Before you transition your body chemistry to keto, any kind of fasting sounds like a strange idea. Once you produce ketones, your appetite decreases. My diarrhea patients have an unknown injury inside their guts. That lining needs to heal. The answer? Rest. In other words, intermittent fasting. Fasting is a universal remedy for many medical problems. When I suggest this to patients, they often resist due to fear of going without food. To help them begin to consider the option, I remind them that animals instinctively fast when they are ill. Rest your guts to allow time for healing. Stop eating.

The ancient Greek physician Hippocrates, regarded as the father of medicine, said this about fasting, "Everyone has a doctor in him; we just have to help him in his work. The natural healing force within each one of us is the greatest force in getting well. To eat when you are sick, is to feed your sickness."

POUNDING HEART

ONSET: Day 2-3.
DURATION: Depends upon the cause, usually a week if caused by de-hydration.

When your heart races inside your chest, a feeling of terror takes over your mind-even if you are a doctor. Your fear is justified. A pounding heart can be a warning of impending death. It signals us to pay attention. If your heart begins to thump inside your chest during ketosis transition, pay attention. Your body is warning you of something.

The most common reason for this symptom is the dehydration mentioned previously. Dehydration forces your heart to pump fast and strong. Fix this problem quickly by drinking salted water! Keep doing this until the heart pounding goes away.

If you have a history of heart arrhythmia, consult your doctor before you go on a keto diet. If your heart is pounding because of an abnormal rhythm, you can drown yourself in salted water making things worse for your heart.

BAD BREATH
ONSET: When you begin making ketones.
DURATION: Until Keto-Adapted

To recap, when your body uses ketones, it releases extra units of this compound as acetone through your breath. It's a dead giveaway you're burning fat for fuel. Acetone smells weird causing metallic- or fruity-scented breath. Surprisingly, many don't experience this problem at all. Others only have acetone breath for a few days. While others can smell the ketones coming out of their sweat and their breath for months on end.

For most people, bad breath lasts for about a month as they adapt to ketosis. The odor usually improves over time as blood ketone levels stabilize in the second or third week.

Remember: acetone ends up in your breath when lots of extra ketones circulate in your blood. When first transitioning to ketosis, your blood can fill with an excessive amount of ketones waiting their turn to be used as fuel. As your cells 'remember' how to use this kind of fuel, there are less excess compounds that can be turned into acetone. Gradually, your body burns ketones as fast as you make them. With less excess ketones, your breath won't stink of acetone.

To deal with acetone breath, try the following:

#1: Get your teeth checked. I found it helpful to remind patients that we evolved using ketones. The human race did not evolve eating starches and sugars. Today's diet fills your mouth with a sugar-bath. This leaves your teeth with tiny pockets where sugar feeds bacteria and other microbes. These hidden cavities allow smelly bacteria to flourish. Cavities and their bacteria are the sources of the long-standing bad breath associated with ketosis.

Get your teeth checked.

Please note that the longer you bathe your teeth in ketones, the stronger and healthier they get. Your ancestors kept their teeth for a lifetime by constantly circulating ketones in their blood and spit. Thanks to their high-fat diet, this continued exposure to ketones strengthened their teeth while fighting the bacteria living in their mouths.

#2: Drink enough water. Dehydration leaves your mouth dry. Mouth dryness concentrates the power of the bacteria living in your oral cavity. Proper hydration flushes and constantly washes your mouth while also diluting the places where bacteria live.

Also, when you drink enough water, you flush ketones from your blood into your urine. You only breathe out acetone when your blood is overflowing with extra ketones. Staying properly hydrated allows your body to get rid of extra ketones through your kidneys. This takes the pressure off your lungs to process ketones and breathe them off as acetone.

#3: If neither of the options above correct your bad breath, reduce the degree of ketosis in your system. Take your pee stick from bright pink to a lighter pink. Ketone production happens in different degrees. The more you produce, the more ketones build up in your blood.

Modulate your ketone level by eating a few more carbs daily. Weight loss won't be as quick, but if the bad breath continues to bother you, eating extra carbs will ensure your blood ketone levels are low enough to avoid acetone breath.

For patients of mine who struggle with bad breath while trying to lose weight through ketosis, I recommend intermittent fasting. I advise them to reach for a 36-hour-fast one time a week. This longer fast in combination with a few more carbs during the other five days of the week slows down weight loss, but reduces acetone breathe.

GOUT

ONSET: 2-4 weeks into ketosis
DURATION: When your rapid weight loss stops

If you've ever had a gout attack, pay attention to this section. Gout happens when waste products crystallize within the body's joints and produce pain when those crystals start to move.

Ketosis significantly reduces your body's inflammation. This causes your body to adjust. One of those adjustments can involve gout crystals getting dislodged from inside your joints-a gout attack.

Don't let a history of gout stop you from a keto diet. Gout crystals formed because of the food you ate years ago. Diets high in carbohydrates combined with fatty meat sparked the problem in your joints. When you switch to a high-fat-low-carb diet, the inflammation drops and the process begins to reverse. As the crystals dissolve, the burden on your joints lessens. But the moment too many crystals move at once, you may spark a gout attack.

Not everybody with a history of gout suffers a flare on this diet. If you've had attacks in your past, you need this lifestyle change more than others. Those crystals hiding in your joints are just a barometer-an indicator-of all the things that have slowly gone wrong deep inside your system. Your high-carb, high-insulin lifestyle has led to gout. Believe it or not, gout crystals are produced by the body as a quick fix. The body stuffs joints full of these extra crystals for storage to prevent your blood from becoming toxic with excess uric acid.

Your body will store these crystals into every joint possible, unless somehow you tip the scales back the other direction. Bathing your system in ketones will reduce insulin and inflammation. This process also dissolves gout crystals. The process of melting such buildup can result in a painful gout flare.

Antidote: Keep your probenecid or your colchicine around. And... of course, stay hydrated.

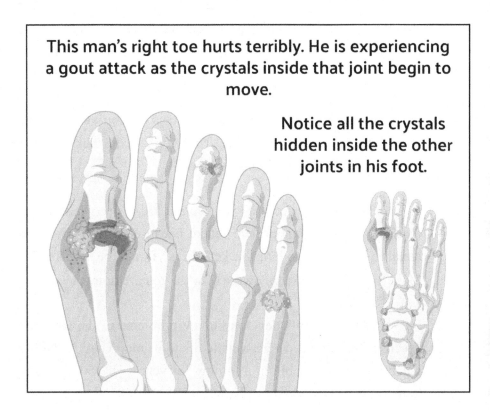

This man's right toe hurts terribly. He is experiencing a gout attack as the crystals inside that joint begin to move.

Notice all the crystals hidden inside the other joints in his foot.

KIDNEY STONES

OBJECTION #6: "Doc, I can't do Keto, I have bad kidneys."

Before I go through kidney stones, let me set one thing straight. If you have kidney problems and have been told that you can't go keto because you need to avoid a high-protein diet, keep in mind this fact: a keto lifestyle is not high in protein. Instead, it is high in fat. Don't confuse the two. Additionally, eating too much protein will kick you out of ketosis. If you are in ketosis, your kidneys are not in danger. The worry that ketosis isn't for patients with kidney problems is a myth.

The bottom line? If you have a kidney problem and are required to limit your protein intake because your kidneys can't handle too much protein, the keto lifestyle can be safe for you. Make your kidney doctor aware of what you are doing.

Many patients develop kidney problems in the first place because they've been overweight for too long. They've had too much insulin or too big of a tummy for years. They've had long-term high blood pressure. These are the problems that destroy kidneys. Most patients with kidney problems don't know they have a kidney problem. Lab tests show they've lost 30% or 40% or even 50% of their kidney function and they didn't have a clue.

Your kidney may be damaged from too many years of high blood pressure, diabetes or pre-diabetes, or plain old obesity. If you have any of these conditions, one of the best things you can do for your kidneys is to get rid of your body's inflammation by cutting out carbs. Let your kidneys flourish in the setting of this anti-inflammatory compound. Let ketones nourish, repair and rejuvenate your kidneys. Oh ... and let's not forget the tremendous relief weight loss will provide for your kidneys.

KIDNEY STONES = KIDNEY CRYSTALS

Multiple crystals grow and shrink at all times

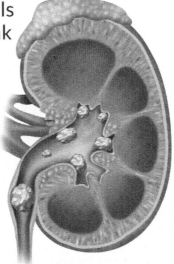

As the crystals change in size, they can dislodge and cause severe pain

Now, on to kidney stones.
ONSET: 2-4 weeks into ketosis
DURATION: When the rapid weight loss stops

Kidney stones should be called kidney crystals. That's what they are: crystals. The formation of these crystal starts with a very tiny chemical attraction between two elements. Your kidney handles a huge volume of these elements every second. If you want to begin making a kidney stone, the first step is to get dehydrated. Run low on water (dehydration) and the concentration of urine in your kidneys shoots way up. This concentrated waste flowing through your kidneys puts these crystallizing elements really close together. Voila! Your first crystal is made.

Next, you add one tiny element to that crystal every time your urine becomes concentrated. As you add one element after another, the crystal grows in size as does its power to attract even more elements. Maybe it takes you 5 years to build that crystal up to a speck. Maybe it takes you 10 years. Unless you 'melt' your kidney stones away, you can grow multiple kidney stones.

Then, one awful day, that big crystal breaks away from the place where it grew. The crystal tumbles through your water works like a boulder. Each tumbler's sharp edges cut and scrape through tissue causing one of life's most excruciatingly painful experiences.

Making kidney stones is painless. No one can feel those tiny changes inside your kidney as the stone grows. If you want to grow those stones faster, add insulin to the system. A high insulin state leads to several changes that are GREAT for growing kidney stones.

If we use a super advanced imaging system to look into the kidneys of adults, almost everyone has tiny little kidney stones. They are growing and shrinking all the time. The stones are either adding crystals or slowly melting away. This is constantly happening.

If your kidney is bathed in crystal-growing chemicals, your stones will continue to grow. High sugar levels favor crystal growth. Ketones favor crystal melting. Ketosis shifts the body's chemistry in the opposite direction.

Does this mean ketosis will melt all the stones lurking in your kidneys?

Not quite.

The good news: ketosis' chemistry shift ensures your kidneys' existing crystals stop growing. Indeed, some of those crystals can disappear over time.

The bad news: Your stone may dislodge before it dissolves.
How come?

When your body produces ketones, kidney stones' crystals get removed one element at a time. We don't get to choose which order the elements peel off of that crystal.

If you have a stone that has been there for years, your new keto-centered blood chemistry may whittle away at the base of the stone. This could set the big stone free to roll down the tubes of the kidney and bladder system. When that stone was securely fixed to the wall of the kidney system, you had no symptoms. If the stone breaks free, boy, oh, boy will you feel it! That crystallized boulder rolls down stream sending shockwaves of pain through your back and groin.

Question: Can ketosis CAUSE you to pass kidney stones?

That's a trick question. It certainly disrupts your body's chemical balance which can lead to your existing stones melting and, in some unlucky situations, passing. Ideally, your body's chemical shift would melt stones one element at a time without dislodging them from their current position. But this is not guaranteed.

ANTIDOTE: Don't cheat! The best way to shake loose a bunch of kidney stones is to go in and out of ketosis a lot. The shift from making the stones to melting the stones unsettles your system.

If you have no stones in your kidney, then you are fine. You won't make new stones while on ketosis. If you have a crop of growing kidney stones and don't know it, beware. If you know you have kidney stones because you have had troubles in the past, you need to commit to this shift in chemistry and stay in ketosis. Pray that the stone melts in an orderly and smooth way. Finally, stay hydrated. A dry kidney is a painful kidney. Never is this more true than when dealing with kidney stones.

MAGNESIUM

ONSET: Days 2-4 into ketosis
DURATION: When you replenish your magnesium level

Most of you reading this book hover on the edge of low magnesium. Almost every patient I see suffers from symptoms triggered by low magnesium. Low magnesium is ubiquitous. Much like sleep deprivation, every modern-day patient should understand what happens to you when this is low.

Magnesium (Mg^{++}), one of your body's most important nutrients, activates hundreds of enzymes, stabilizes your cellular structure, and triggers many of your cell proteins to do their job. Magnesium is a required salt. You get it from your food. In turn, your food gets it from the soil. The marked decline in soil magnesium content in many parts of the world yields plants lacking this super important mineral. As with any food chain, when the lowest link on the chain struggles to access needed minerals, the rest of us higher on the chain suffer too.

Low magnesium symptoms include headaches, dizziness, confusion, mental cloudiness (also called brain fog), nervousness, and tingling in your hands and feet.

When Mg^{++} falls below the threshold needed for your nerves to properly send signals, patients most commonly complain about muscle cramping. Truth be told, my patients have had multiple symptoms before their muscles cramped. They did not associate those symptoms to low magnesium. When I discuss muscles cramps, patients usually think of a charlie-horse or a crick in their neck. But other common symptoms of a cramping muscle include a headache in the back of your head, or near your temples. Symptoms can also involve a deep tummy pain due to your bladder or bowel muscles cramping. You might even experience heart arrhythmia or chest pain from the cramping of your heart muscle. All these are common symptoms that can crop up for people with low magnesium.

Dropping magnesium levels cause your brain processing to slow down and even 'twitch.' These symptoms commonly take the form of depression or anxiety.

These frequent, yet unexpected symptoms of low magnesium, happen when you get diarrhea. You lose a lot of magnesium all at once through your loose stools. Similarly, as you shift your body chemistry from the Standard American Diet to a Ketosis Diet the swift shift in fluids lowers your magnesium. Within hours of that drop, patients complain of a profound sadness or irritability. They will say the diet makes them crabby or lose focus. That night, a startling jerk in their foot pulls them right out

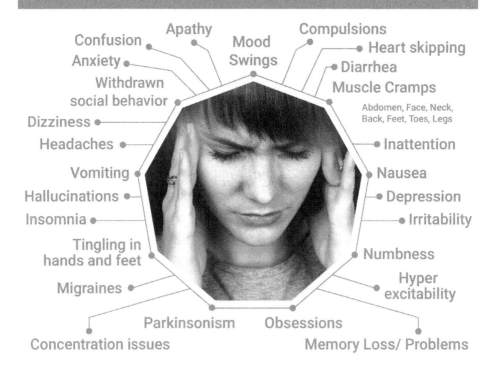

Symptoms of Low Magnesium

Confusion
Apathy
Mood Swings
Compulsions
Heart skipping
Anxiety
Diarrhea
Withdrawn social behavior
Muscle Cramps
Abdomen, Face, Neck, Back, Feet, Toes, Legs
Dizziness
Headaches
Inattention
Vomiting
Nausea
Hallucinations
Depression
Insomnia
Irritability
Tingling in hands and feet
Numbness
Migraines
Hyper excitability
Parkinsonism
Obsessions
Concentration issues
Memory Loss/ Problems

of their slumber. That's usually when they consider magnesium as the culprit.

ANTIDOTE: Naturally it is to replace magnesium. Sounds simple enough, right? However, adding a large dose of magnesium to your gut causes diarrhea. One dose of milk of magnesia flushes constipation away. Scamming vitamin suppliers have a tough time fooling consumers with even the most basic understanding of magnesium: If the magnesium supplement you're taking does not cause your tummy to rumble, it's probably a scam product.

Telling you to eat high magnesium foods sounds like good advice at first glance. But this advice falls short if the foods themselves are no longer reliable in their magnesium content due to poor soil nutrients across the globe.

I recommend a different option. Use your skin. Yes, that's right. Use your body's largest organ to absorb magnesium.

My favorite recommendation is to write the following prescription: Add 6 cups of Magnesium Chloride Salt to hot bath water. Soak for 40 minutes twice weekly.

Not only does this help you absorb magnesium, it also adds some much-needed relaxation time to your schedule. Epsom Salt, Magnesium Sulfate Salt, is also used for soaking magnesium baths. From my experience, Magnesium Chloride baths deliver more intensive and complete relief from magnesium deficiency symptoms.

Other options include magnesium salt-enriched creams or oils. Although not nearly as rewarding as a 40 minute bath, these topical applications do a good job relieving symptoms when applied routinely.

OBJECTION #7: "Low carb diets cause high cholesterol"

That answer is partly true. But the cholesterol that goes up is actually your good (HDL) cholesterol. To make this happen, you have to decrease and eventually remove carbohydrates from your diet. Cut out carbs and watch triglycerides drop.

Raising your good cholesterol and dropping your triglyceride levels leads to a healthier heart. How come? Cutting down on carbs lowers inflammation for your system.

Bad (LDL) cholesterol is another story. Cholesterol was sold to us as a heart disease predictor. The cholesterol you eat is a fraction of what you make inside your body. Your liver and other cells make cholesterol to maintain your tissues. It is a crucial repair substance needed for correcting cellular damage.

Cholesterol is also the starting compound for making important hormones such as estrogen, testosterone, progesterone, cortisol, and aldosterone. This compound is an integral part of your brain and is crucial for proper nerve cell function. Without cholesterol, the human body doesn't work.

Actually, our body makes extra cholesterol when it detects something needs repairing.

Elevated cholesterol indicates the presence of inflammation and tissue damage. Cholesterol can warn us of an underlying problem of inflammation.

A high fat low carb diet lowers both inflammation and blood cholesterol levels. Reread that sentence again. It's worth repeating. A high fat low carb diet lowers both inflammation and blood cholesterol levels.

HIGH CARBOHYDRATE DIET　　　**HIGH FAT DIET**

Both fasting serum from the same patient.

The fat-filled plasma was obtained during the high-carbohydrate eating.

The clear plasma during the high-fat regime.

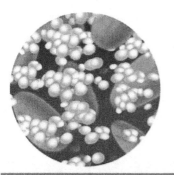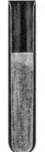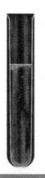

CARBOHYDRATE-INDUCED AND FAT-INDUCED LIPEMIA
AHRENS ET AL.
Transactions of Association of American Physicians 1961

Take a look at these 2 blood samples from the <u>same patient</u>. This is a 1961 report from the Association of American Physicians. They placed patients on a high carbohydrate diet and tested their fasting plasma (the colorless fluid part of your blood.) They then placed the same patients on several weeks of a high fat diet with low carbohydrates. After weeks of each diet, they tested the patient's fasting plasma.

The high carbohydrate diet filled the plasma sample with cholesterol's white, fatty globules. (Notice the test tube on the left.)

However, plasma from the high fat, low carb diet of the same patient yielded a clear serum with little to no suspended fat. (The test tube on the right.)

Atherosclerosis can be arrested after two years on a keto-genic diet. This is consistent with my patients' clinical experience. The key part of this equation is that you MUST lower your carbs while eating high fat. Without honoring both of those rules at the same time, you are headed for disaster.

Don't play around.

Be sure you prove to yourself and the medical world that you are indeed producing ketones.

Check regularly.

Chapter 19

Lessons from Dr. Bosworth:

BEGINNERS' GROCERIES

This is a dirty trick. If you opened this book and wanted to rush to the store and buy keto diet-friendly foods, STOP.

Please don't go grocery shopping until you have successfully done the 'How Do I Start' chapter.

For the rest of you, use this food collection to restock your pantry. Remember when I asked you to, "PAUSE." This list is what I would ask you to take with you to the grocery store after you paused.

Keep a supply of the following:

FROZEN FOODS:
Broccoli
Cauliflower
Peppers
Onions (dried is better than frozen)

Okra

Spinach

Kale

Frozen blackberries (This is the only fruit on the list.)

FRESH FOODS

A whole head of cabbage

Avocados

When first going keto, frozen vegetables kept me on the keto wagon many times. They helped me avoid cheating when I did not have time to go to the grocery store or chop fresh vegetables. As my palate changed, I found having a head of cabbage in the fridge was far more rewarding to eat than the frozen veggies. Cabbage did not spoil in the fridge and rewarded my craving for a fresh taste. Alternatively, tossing sliced cabbage with melted butter and garlic and placing it under the broiler made for a fast, tasty addition to meals.

Avocados and I have had a love-hate relationship. I love the taste when they are fresh. I will salt a ripe avocado and eat it right out of its skin. But in my neck of the woods they are far too costly to open one up and find it was last week's good idea. Use this trick when you open an avocado and find it starting to spoil. Scoop the avocado out into a ziplock bag and place in the freezer. Frozen avocados added to heavy whipping cream or coconut cream are the foundation to dozens of frozen fat-bomb recipes. I have added peanut butter powder, some macadamia nuts, and a hint of stevia to the blender for the perfect keto fix.

I had several spices and herbs in my cupboard before I began keto, but they had been in those same spice shakers for a half dozen years. This shift in food fuel sent me recipe hunting for great-tasting keto friendly foods. My initial failure to produce ketones was in large part due to the hidden carbs in the food I had grown accustomed to. Once I finally made a few ketones, I only trusted the foods I personally prepared in my kitchen. This list of flavors took my kitchen experiments to the next level.

Rosemary

Ginger

Basil (Buy a potted plant of basil. The extreme taste difference between fresh basil and dried basil amazes my tongue every time.)

Oregano

Italian Seasoning

Cajun Seasoning

Black Pepper

Pink Salt

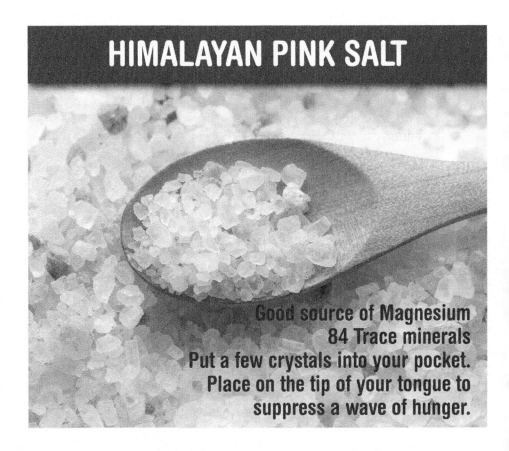

HIMALAYAN PINK SALT

Good source of Magnesium
84 Trace minerals
Put a few crystals into your pocket.
Place on the tip of your tongue to
suppress a wave of hunger.

After two weeks of ketosis, and a few nights of leg cramps, I found every possible way to improve my magnesium. Salt baths corrected many of my symptoms. However, the addition of Himalayan Pink Salt to all my foods and a few crystals in my pocket helped prevent low magnesium problems or suffering sleepless nights.

Every keto kitchen must have an abundance of eggs, real butter, and heavy whipping cream. Nearly every keto treats recipe includes these ingredients. Cans of Coconut Cream are a new normal for my pantry. In unexpected moments when my whipping cream carton runs empty, coconut cream is there to rescue my recipes. I store one can in the fridge to harden up the fat enough so I can pour off the coconut water. Fast, tasty and spoilage-resistant.

Lemon / Lime Juice
Cinnamon
Vanilla Extract
Cacao Powder (not cocoa powder)
Coconut Cream (3-4 cans)
Pili nuts
Macadamia Nuts
Chia Seeds
Almond Butter
Almonds

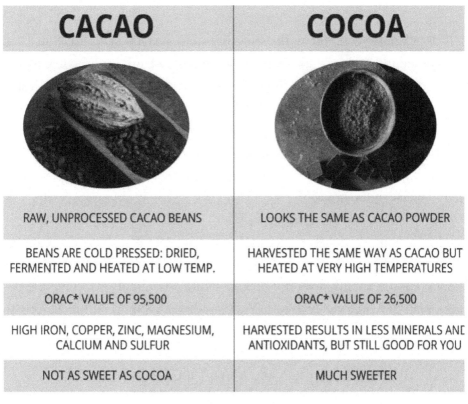

CACAO	COCOA
RAW, UNPROCESSED CACAO BEANS	LOOKS THE SAME AS CACAO POWDER
BEANS ARE COLD PRESSED: DRIED, FERMENTED AND HEATED AT LOW TEMP.	HARVESTED THE SAME WAY AS CACAO BUT HEATED AT VERY HIGH TEMPERATURES
ORAC* VALUE OF 95,500	ORAC* VALUE OF 26,500
HIGH IRON, COPPER, ZINC, MAGNESIUM, CALCIUM AND SULFUR	HARVESTED RESULTS IN LESS MINERALS AND ANTIOXIDANTS, BUT STILL GOOD FOR YOU
NOT AS SWEET AS COCOA	MUCH SWEETER

*METHOD OF MEASURING ANTIOXIDANT POWER

FAT FACTS

Fats and oils fall into three major groups: saturated, monounsaturated, and polyunsaturated.

• Saturated fats (SFA) are solid at room temperature. Examples: lard, butter, and coconut oil. These fats are the most chemically stable and least inflammatory.

• Monounsaturated fats (MUFA) include beef tallow, olive oil, avocado oil, macadamia oil, and hazelnut oil.

• Polyunsaturated fats (PUFA) are the least stable of all fats. They are prone to rancidity and are easily affected by heat and light. PUFA come in two types: omega-6 and omega-3. Omega-6 fats tend to be more inflammatory. Somewhat less inflammatory are the ever popular omega-3 fats found in fish oil and fatty fish.

Choose your fat with your digestive system in mind. Saturated and monounsaturated fats such as butter, macadamia nuts, coconut oil, olive oil, avocado oil, and egg yolks are easier on your stomach. Many people cannot handle eating large amounts of polyunsaturated fats. Omega-6 PUFA vegetable oils such as soybean, sunflower, safflower, corn, and canola oils are no longer found in my cupboards. Neither are many products containing these oils such as commercially processed mayonnaise and margarine.

When I coach patients on what type of fat to buy, I encourage them to find food they like. I spend a great deal of time reassuring patients that the enemy does not lurk in saturated animal-fats. Save the bacon fat to fry up your broccoli. YUM! When shopping add these oils to your cart:

MCT Oil Powder (Be sure it says C8:C10)
Coconut Oil
Butter
Olive Oil

Salty treats are a MUST on this diet. Since transitioning to this diet, I've added these two items to my cupboard.

Olives in Oil
Muffuletta Olive Salad (in a jar). Never heard of this? Just buy it. When you get tired of plain eggs, add this. It makes all the difference.

Sugar substitutes are not recommended long term. However, for the beginner it certainly provides a bridge to use instead of sugar. Ketone success happens when these are removed from your life. Use with caution:

Stevia

Truvia [Erythritol (a sugar alcohol) + Rebaudioside A (a sweet compound isolated from the stevia plant)]

Monk Fruit

The rest of the list . . .

Cream Cheese

Heavy Whipping Cream

Mayonnaise from Avocado Oil

Sardines in Oil (Don't complain until you have tried them.)

Liverwurst (Don't freak out. Just try it.)

Coffee

Tea

Mineral Water

Kombucha

OBJECTION #8: "What about exercise? I am training for a marathon, and use carbs, carbs, carbs for my fuel."

First of all, good for you for running a marathon. These people are freaks of nature. To run 26 miles is one thing; to run it again and again striving for your personal best is inspirational.

Endurance athletes pay lots of attention to their food-energy. If they run out of usable energy at the end of their race, bad things happen.

The next time your community is hosting a marathon, volunteer to hand out water or guard an intersection in the last mile of the race. Watch what happens to some of the ill-prepared athletes as they push themselves at the end of the race.

'Bonking' is the term for running out of fuel during an endurance race. Specifically, the fuel for their brain is missing. If they are traditional athletes, their bodies are carb-fueled. Their glucose fuel source must be replenished again and again throughout the race. They burn through their "pine-needles" wickedly fast with all the energy needed to race. This produces a delicate situation once they have used up all their stored sugars in the form of glycogen. They need to throw the proper amount of 'pine needles' into their furnaces to keep racing. If they run out of glucose, they 'bonk.' Their brain shuts down because it is totally glucose-dependent.

Even a lean athlete with under 15% body fat can carry more than 50,000 kilocalories in their fat. These calories are useless to them because their system is not adapted to burning fat for fuel. And let me tell you, the last mile of a 100 mile race is not the time to be asking your body to figure out ketosis. After several hours of intense exercise, an athlete running out of available glucose will describe their 'bonk' as a strange experience where a dramatic loss in performance, a profound sudden depression and intense food cravings coincide. Observers may notice the athlete shake and quiver with chills. They lose control of their bowels or bladder. They stumble as if drunk while their brain scrambles to find any morsel of glucose lingering around.

On the other hand, fat-fueled endurance athletes, have the flexibility to choose their fuel sources. If they practiced fueling from fat for weeks before their race, they have a distinct advantage. Their brain cells can use either fuel. If their body gets low on fuel, they can add some glucose and use it. But if they run out of glucose, their keto-adapted cells activate the part of their furnaces that burn fat instead of carbs. This transition happens in a flash if they are keto-adapted. They don't poop their pants. They don't 'bonk,' unless they suffer from the very rare problem of running out of fat.

The bonking athlete is much like a diesel-powered truck that runs out of fuel while hauling a tank filled with gasoline. There is gasoline fuel in his tank, but diesel engines are not equipped to use gasoline.

Fat-fueled, low-carb endurance athletes aren't just running races, they are winning at record breaking times. Nothing grabs the attention of competitive endurance athletes, like titles. These athletes are tossing out the carb-dense foods and chewing on fat for their fuel. Just think how much time gets shaved off a race if they don't have to pause for a bathroom break ten times in the race's last stretch.

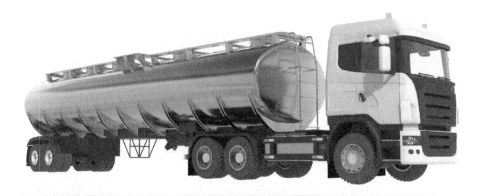

When an athlete "hits the wall" or "bonks" it is like a tanker truck hauling gasoline running out of diesel fuel.

The tanker truck holds a bunch of fuel in his cargo, but the diesel engine is not equipped to use that kind of fuel.

WARNING TO ATHLETES: If you switch your fuel from carbs to a fat-fueled system plan on a few weeks of decreased performance before you reap the benefits. Don't flip to this the week before your big race. Review the chapter on the 5 phases of keto adaptation. Take special notice of when your muscles and brain reach optimal ketone processing proficiency. To gain the advantage of powering your body from either fuel, you need 4-6 weeks of consistent ketosis before you race.

But what does this all mean for the rest of us?

Burning fat for fuel allows a steady production of ketones. Hunger simply disappears. Hunger comes from blood sugars that swing up and down. From high to low. High. Low. High. Low. When the body's fuel source is stable instead of bouncing up and down, food cravings disappear. More importantly, inflammation within your body decreases each week you produce ketones.

COMPARE 100 GRAMS OF FOOD					
FOOD 100 GRAMS	Water	Fat	Carbs	Protein	TOTAL GRAMS
SUGAR	0	0	100	0	100
OLIVE OIL	0	100	0	0	100
EGGS	76	10	1	13	100
LARD	0	100	0	0	100
BUTTER	18	81	0	1	100
HEAVY CREAM	58	37	3	2	100
FETA	61	21	4	14	100
STEAK	71	7	0	21	100
SARDINES	64	11	0	25	100
LIVERWURST	54	28	3	15	100
BROCCOLI	90	0	7	3	100

Chapter 20

Lessons from Dr. Bosworth:
INTERMITTENT FASTING

INTERMITTENT FASTING: NOT A LOW CALORIE DIET. Please, do not confuse my support of intermittent fasting with support for starving. Let me be clear: NO STARVING ALLOWED!

Reduced calorie diets are a no-no. Intermittent Fasting (IF) knocks the socks off of a Low Calorie or Reduced Calorie diet. Indeed, I would say they are the OPPOSITE of each other. Intermittent fasting shifts your chemistry in the opposite direction of the low calorie diets.

A calorie-reduced diet would be more accurately called a torture diet. No matter its name, it triggers your chemistry to store fat. This low calorie setting takes your food and squirrels it away into cells designated to store energy. If you want a body chemistry that locks your energy efficiently into your fat cells, go on a reduced calorie diet. Every study regarding reduced calorie diets has proven this over and over again.

Notice that I have not mentioned carbohydrates or fat. When scouring through every reduced calorie diet, notice that the instructors of these diets select food with the fewest calories. Fats add the most calories per bite, therefore are sparingly selected for these diets. When the dietician adds fat to the list of foods, suddenly their low calorie diet is no longer low in calories.

Look at the diet comparison graph showing calories along the bottom and the carbohydrates along the left side.

For example, one very low calorie diet recommends a total daily intake of 800 kilocalories (kcal) in the form of liquids or protein bar supplements. The results? After several weeks, people on this diet might see significant weight loss. However, their bodies are in crisis. Their system is stressed, and you can measure their stress hormones to prove it. They don't sleep well. They feel tired, crabby, and count down to the day they can start eating again. Sadly, their metabolism suffered the greatest damage. During the 8 weeks of their diet ordeal, their body remains in the 'store all that you can find' mode. When they resume eating, watch out. BOOOM! The calories will be sucked into storage never to be released again.

Why does the body react this way?

The body registered a trickle of incoming fuel and those limited resources transmitted a message that you are 'about to face starvation.' The key word is 'about.' Never do they actually enter a time of absent calories. Evolution has taught each of your cells that when food gets this scarce, they need to store calories away because there's a famine coming. People on starvation or reduced calorie diets are only a few hundred calories away from a biochemical state where their cells say the opposite message.

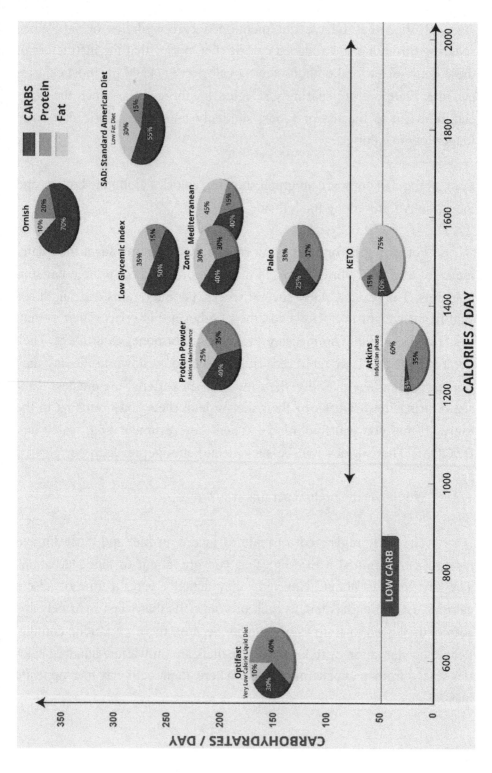

Take away those final calories and the message changes to 'We are in a famine, release calories from storage. We need to survive by using all resources from within our body.'

By consuming low calories instead of zero calories, your body chemistry never fully shifts to fasting mode. You miss out on the advantages of fasting.

A low-calorie diet gradually slows down your metabolism. Your body prepares for what is to come by conserving every possible calorie. Your cells' internal furnace also helps by reducing the energy burned in the mitochondria throughout the body. Translation: you're tired.

This 'pre-fasting' state sabotages even the most diligent people. In this biochemical state, you torture your body with a grumbling hunger, a nervous irritability, as well as an unsettled feeling of impending stress. How does your body do this? In a word, it's your chemistry.

Low-calorie diets provide the ideal chemistry to keep fat inside your fat cells. The longer you stick to your torture-based-diet, the greater the damage to your metabolic motor. Put simply, you're caught in a race to the bottom!

Eventually, you will eat normally again. I've had patients stay on these low calorie diets for months, even years and their metabolism plummeted to as little as 600 calories a day! At that level, it's so easy for them to gain weight. Every tiny bit of food they eat after the first 600 calories goes right into their fat storage. It stays there forever! Locked! The body compensates for all the lost time spent begging for more calories by storing anything extra. That chemical signal remains active for weeks after they start eating again. It's as if their body does not trust that the food will remain available. In my clinic, it takes 6-12 weeks to fix that broken metabolism.

To sum up, if you go on a calorie reduced diet :
Your metabolism slows down.
You are hungry all the time.
You reverse any weight loss process because you are fighting against your own hormones.

Now you might ask "How the heck is a reduced calorie diet different from fasting?"

Strangely, the difference when measured by calorie intake is only a few hundred calories apart, but the divergent biochemical effects could not be more pronounced.

Fasting chemistry is an extension of ketogenic chemistry. Both fasting-based chemistry and ketosis-based chemistry produce the opposite effects of a low-calorie-setting. Completely halting your intake of calories switches ON your body's ketone production system.

I explain it to my patients this way: In a low-calorie-chemical state, those few calories tell your body that you're actually going to respond to the hunger and eat. Your body receives the signal that there's food around-just not very much. Your body gets the command to hold on to any calories it comes across, and even sends some irritable, aggressive signals to your brain to grab food! Your body then stores many of those calories for the perceived impending famine.

When you're fasting, your body gets the very clear message that there is no food. You are on your own to survive until food becomes available again. The chemistry and hormones hear ONE MESSAGE: No food. The chemical message is: 'Don't die between now and the next meal. Use your stored energy.' This signal is clear and effective. Within 12 hours, your body chemistry begins to shift. This biochemical signal is loudest and clearest after 72 hours of fasting. Chemical signals surge throughout your body instructing cells to burn calories from your energy reserves-your stored fat!

Ketosis and fasting are on the same spectrum of body chemistry. Of course, fasting features a more intense chemical setting compared to ketosis.

Intermittent fasting sends a very clear and distinct chemical message to your body to shift and adapt to no calories for the next 12, 24, or 36 hours-however long you remain fasting. When you eat, do not wreck that chemical shift with carbohydrates or excess protein. Instead, adopt a high-fat ketosis diet. Doing so keeps your insulin levels low and allows your cells access to your body's stored calories-your fat deposits if needed..

Studies indicate that calorie-reduction body chemistry leads to a disastrous metabolic mess. This happens Every. Single. Time. A host of studies have shown when you reduce calories, the body slips into slower metabolism. Also your body instinctively stores calories in preparation for starvation. It stores all that energy and awaits the 'drought' of calories certainly coming soon. When we restrict, instead of stopping calorie intake, we get stuck in that pre-starving (pre-fasting) chemistry.

Look carefully at this chart documenting the progress of a person losing fifty pounds of fat. Before switching to ketosis, she had whittled her metabolism down to 800 calories per day. She needed 800 measly calories to keep her alive. If she ate exactly 800 per day, her system

KETO PATIENT 50 POUND- WEIGHT LOSS OVER 54 WEEKS.					
	PRE-KETO	INDUCTION	ADAPTING	KETO-ADAPTED	MAINTAIN
		Week 1	Weeks 2-13	Weeks 14-53	Weeks 54+
Weight	210	200	180	160	150
Daily Calories Consumed	**800**	**1400**	**1800**	**2150**	**2200**
Total Calories Used in a Day	**800**	**2800**	**2600**	**2400**	**2200**
Daily Carb Grams	130	20	25-30	30-40	55
Pounds of **Fat** Weight Lost Every Week	0	0 All 20 lbs = water weight lost while metabolism boosts.	1.7 Best Fat Loss	0.5 Continued, steady Fat Loss	0

would use those 800 calories to stay alive and signal every mitochondria to slow down. 'Use less energy.'

Tomorrow her body would need only 799 calories to stay alive. If she ate 130 carbohydrates through her low calorie/low fat diet but accidentally ate one extra bite pushing her total to 820 calories, all 20 of those extra calories would go into storage. She would get fatter. Her body followed the rules by putting every extra calorie into her fat cells. In our example anything over 800 calories is extra because she is in 'pre-starvation' mode. Her body protected her by storing all extra calories above her body's energy expenditure, or the base amount of energy to keep her alive.

In the chart, she switches to a ketogenic diet which sparked a chemistry shift that flushed out her extra water and began the slow rehabilitation of her broken metabolism. The first twenty pounds she lost came from getting rid of all that extra water.

Twenty five days after she started, her body fully adapted to using fat as her fuel. Notice her 'Expenditure' row. This refers to how much energy it takes to fuel her body each day. Think back to your furnaces. In the 800 calorie setting, her furnaces were all but shut down. Any remaining furnaces all burned her carb-based fuel- those 'pine needles' that burn hot and fast. Initially she argued with me saying, "But Doc, I am on a high protein diet." She failed to grasp that she forced most of those proteins into carb-fuel because of her pre-starvation chemistry.

The difference between an 800 calorie energy expenditure and a 2800 calorie expenditure sparked a lightning bolt throughout her body. Her 800 calorie-fueled-system made her look and feel wilted-complete with thin hair, dull skin and a brain that limps from one task to the next. During my first visit with her, I noticed her muffled and slurred speech- symptoms of a swollen, toxic, sugar-fed brain.

The 2800-calorie-eating took two weeks to awaken her lifeless mitochondria and lit a fire-cracker to her metabolism. How did I know her metabolism was so high? It didn't take a medical degree to figure that out. Everyone saw it. Her energy was contagious.

She lost 70 pounds over that year. It is worth noting that the chart shows her first 50 pounds. The final 20 pounds came when she lowered her carbs back to about 30 grams per day. Her history of 'energy-storing chemistry' was very sensitive to carbohydrates. The slightest increase in carbs and her system slipped into making insulin and locking her fat cells closed.

OBJECTION # 9 "Wait. Why was she eating 30 carbs per day? Doesn't this violate the 20-gram-rule?"

She simply measured her blood ketones and glucose. She studied herself. When she ate more than 50 carbs per day, her blood ketones were rarely in ketosis (any reading greater than 0.5mM.) When she stayed at 20 carbs per day, she was always in ketosis but found herself giving in to temptation. She gradually increased her carb intake to 30 grams per day where she was still in ketosis, yet able to eat enough carbs to say no to the foods she should not eat.

This diet is a measurable chemistry equation. Measure your chemistry to prove to yourself what is happening with your system. Fit your food intake into the equation to get the desired effect.

By the end of that year, she had radiant skin tone, healthy new hair growth, and abundant energy. The best victory in her ketogenic transition is that this woman now has the metabolism that will enable her to fall off the keto wagon every once in awhile. If she overeats and stops producing ketones, she still has a built-in motor to reverse any imbalance before her cheating will have a chance to produce much weight gain.

When asked what the key to her success was she replied, "Testing my ketones every day. I had to be honest with myself. I became the ketone pee stick lady at work. I had to keep proving to myself that I was eating right. Lots of friends and family thought I was nuts for eating so much fat. Ketone sticks helped me to know I was doing this correctly and scientifically. Everyday, I peed on a stick. That made all the difference."

CLINCHER:

Calorie reduction increases your hunger and decreases your metabolism.

Intermittent fasting does the opposite. It decreases your appetite while stimulating your metabolism-all while burning your stored fat.

Chapter 21

Grandma Rose: A 40 DAY FAST INTERRUPTED

For the next two days, I guarded her hospital room. Our goal was forty days of fasting-in secret. Neither of us had the confidence or energy to pull anyone else onto our bandwagon. In the quiet darkness of the hospital room, we planned our next steps.

The next morning, her medical team offered her carb-filled hospital food. To us, this represented the enemy. Carbs a.k.a. sugar. Sugar a.k.a. The Devil.

Her orders in the chart reflected their plan to slowly introduce foods back to her diet. The trays of jello and ice cream and pudding came. Smiles all around. The nurses left and her food went straight down the toilet. FLUSH!

We secretly flushed ALL her hospital food, hiding any evidence of our lies.

Meanwhile, I snuck her in the 'good stuff.' BONE BROTH.

Had you asked me to read this story a year prior, I would have said this woman might be a medical doctor, but she is going to kill her mother.

Several times throughout the prior months, I had read about keto folks using bone broth for their fasts. Fasting remained this out-of-reach idea before now. Every time I encountered information about these longer fasts, I skimmed over them confident I would never need that information. The night her abscesses drained, I crouched in the dimness of her hospital hallway scrolling back to find all the missed information.

There were some goofy rules about useless bone broth versus a nutrient-dense version. Expecting to never taste it, let alone live off it for over a month, I hadn't even read the information. In the hospital shadows, I had learned that bone broth was not quite the salted water I had imagined. In contrast, this nutrient-dense concoction was a spoonful of gold.

The difference began with the bones. Lots of little bones, such as those from chickens or knuckle bones from cows, provided greater surface area for bone marrow. The marrow, found inside the hollow part of a bone, filled each bite with Mary Poppins magic. Each bite is packed with nutrients. If all she ate for 40 days was bone marrow broth, she had a chance of making it. And by 'making it' I meant living-versus dying.

At that moment, her swollen, blocked-off, inflamed, infected intestines had created a tunnel from the insides of her guts connecting those engorged abscesses. This detour linked her unused food to the top of her vagina. This fragile mess of a tunnel needed as little of a job as possible.

Several teaspoons of dense nutrients would enter into her stomach and our hope was that all but a speck of that nutrients would be absorbed before arriving at her detour tunnel.

THE GOOD STUFF: How can you tell 'good' bone broth from the worthless version? Good broth remained in gel form at room temperature. This is the quick and dirty way to prove the broth had enough glucosamine, chondroitin and other marrow proteins to provide the nutrient density Grandma Rose needed. We wanted her home and away from all things hospital.

The doctors promised removal of her IVs once her diet advanced to 'normal.' We avoided the official definition of that word. Nourishment entered her stomach and was absorbed completely before it got to her newly rerouted exit.

I called out to friends on social media: "Mayday! Mayday! NEEDED: Gelatinous Bone Broth for Grandma Rose." Not surprising, no one understood what I was talking about. Bone broth was a foreign term to most who read the message-not even factoring in the additional term 'gelatinous.' I followed up with video education using YouTube. My virtual classroom for fellow Midwestern pioneers sparked an old fashion cook-off.

"Mary, Mary, quite contrary. How does your bone broth gel?"

Grandma Rose fasted for another three days as we awaited the special delivery of bone broth. A complete fast scared me, but she marched through those days like a champion. The IV salted and hydrated her system just right. We celebrated every time we tested her urine ketones: very high levels.

Her first swallow of broth left both of us anxious about a looming reaction. She took one tablespoon full of the salty, warm liquid. And then we waited.

An hour later, she took bite number two.

Still nothing. At the 1/2 cup point, a slight wave of cramps hit her tummy and sliced through our courage. We stopped for that day.

The cramps did not last long. She rested.

Relieved by the lack of trouble, we tried again the following day. Once again, success. She ate a 1/4 of a cup twice that day. Before the end of the second day, we found black specks in the slime of her panty liner. Without food, the slick discharge had all but stopped except for a smear of mucous on her panty liner. It looked like … like thick snot. Sometimes a little blood tinged the pad, but the day after her first bone broth, black specks appeared in the slime.

We stared at the pad in silence, then at one another wondering what we had done.

In unison we said, "pepper." We had seasoned the bone broth with salt and pepper. That 'speck' of remaining nutrients making it out the exit had arrived.

By the fourth day, she drank two servings of hot, salty broth. It worked.

Ten days of fasting and we claimed success. And by we I mean Grandma Rose. My grand ambitions of fasting as long as Grandma Rose melted after the third day.

I had left the hospital dazed with distracted thoughts of Grandma Rose's convoluted pooping system. Caught in my mental fog, I drove through, completely on auto-pilot, and ordered my default cream-filled coffee. I realized I had broken my fast when it was about half gone. Dang!

But not Grandma Rose. She stuck to it! 'Do or Die' helped her stay on course. I wanted to add to her momentum, but she flew solo. Ten days with nothing to eat except small amounts of bone broth and she soared on the winds of her Mary Poppins magic.

The hospital team remained unaware that all sugar and carbs fed her toilet bowl. The unfortunate dietician from the hospital kitchen faced our collective anger when she offered Grandma Rose a chocolate ice cream shake.

Outside of snapping at the dietician, Grandma Rose looked high. Euphoric. Not painkiller kind of high; she was off of those. Her mental zone persisted in a state of exhilaration ratcheting up one notch at a time. Her elation rose higher and higher. One night she could not sleep. Not a wink. Skirting on the edge of some sort of enlightenment, she could not shut down.

My late night, speed-reading about extended fasts warned me about this possibility. The advanced mental performance shows up around day five according to most of the blogs and reports I had read. Indeed, that predictable sleepless night took place, but in Grandma Rose's case it arrived between fasting day eleven and twelve.

The longer the fast went on, the quicker she seemed to heal. Her energy ascended to the highest level she had felt in months. The magic of Mary Poppins, or the power of the Holy Spirit, percolated through her veins.

On fasting day number thirteen, without anyone knowing of her fast, she left the hospital.

Why not tell the hospital team what we were doing?

Well, it was just too much of a hassle. Ketosis seemed too unconventional to share with my colleagues-let alone fasting during times of severe, life-threatening illness. It mattered nothing that national experts and historians alike agreed with me. What mattered was the team in front of me. They did the very best job they knew how. I could not plug the ketogenic education into the minds of the team members caring for Grandma Rose. I could not suggest the science of fasting either. Presenting these options to the medical team would have only created conflict. The additional stress would not have been healthy for Grandma Rose.

The farm provided protection by putting distance between Grandma Rose and the rest of the world. She found strength in the isolation of our old farmhouse.

OBJECTION #10: "If I fast I will break down my own muscles for body fuel."

Not true. The human body wasn't meant to break down it's muscles for fuel. If that were true, we would have never lived through countless famines and long winters in our history as a species. When your body goes without food, it will tap into your fat storage and use it for energy. Sure, in extreme stages of starvation we use our muscles as fuel. But fat gets emptied first. Prove to your naysayers that you're burning fats by showing off your positive ketones results. A positive urine ketone stick says 'I'm wasting unused fuel and energy out my urine. This wasted fuel came from stored fat.' Please, don't be intimidated by the misinformed. The idea that fasting causes you to cannibalize your muscle tissues to use as fuel is simply not true. Mother Nature did a far better job of protecting us than that.

Chapter 22

Lessons from Dr. Bosworth:

THE WONDERFUL MYSTERY OF AUTOPHAGY

Autophagy. The literal translation of this word: 'to eat thyself.'

Autophagy is a hot topic. Yoshinori Ohsumi's 2016 Nobel Prize for Physiology and Medicine converted the medical world's previous whispers and murmurings about autophagy into a full-blown conversation. Ohsumi discovered how our body degrades and recycles its cellular components. Autophagy for short.

Why should you care? This book is supposed to be focused on ketones.

Well, it turns out ketones and autophagy are linked.

Baby Boomers: please pay attention. You endured the most abuse from the medical establishment over the last 40 years. Before it's too late, we in the medical establishment might have a few years to redeem some of the atrocious recommendations that your generation lived through. The science of how your body eats itself is something you should pay attention to.

It may sound weird, but this process of autophagy might be the saving grace to medicine of your era. The science of autophagy surfaced in the nick of time for Boomers.

Bone Broth That Gels Every Single Time

Prep Time: 5 mins   **Cook Time in instant pot:** 4 hours   **Servings:** 8 cups

INGREDIENTS   www.MeatButterEggs.com
* 8 cups water   Measure the water. Do not fill your instant pot to the fill line. It's too much water.
* 2 whole chickens carcasses. Remove the meat and use the leftover bones. Your pot should be as full as you can get it.
* 1 package chicken feet (about 20 feet)
* 1 tsp salt

INSTRUCTIONS
1. Throw bones, chicken feet, salt and water into your pot.
2. Using the soup function on your instapot, set your time to 240 minutes. Make sure your valve is closed.
3. After 4 hours let the instant pot do a natural pressure release to avoid broth spraying all over your kitchen.
4. Strain through a cheesecloth into containers. Eat or let cool before chilling in the refrigerator overnight and then freezing what you won't use up that week.
5. Don't remove the fat off the top. It helps seal the broth and keeps it fresh.

INSTANT POT: This is a modern day pressure cooker. It is safer than the traditional pressure cookers and adds a variety of foods to the list.

BONES: Save the carcsses from rotisserie chicken in the freezer. When you have enough bones to fill your pot, make broth.

CHICKEN FEET: Don't leave out the feet. The collagen comes from the chicken feet. This makes your broth rich, flavorful, and nutritionally dense. Using an instant pot, or a traditional pressure cooker, there is no need blanch, skin or remove the nails. Just throw them all into the pot. There is no difference in taste or appearance.

Autophagy removes debris found inside your body's cells. All those years of poorly fed brain cells, sleep deprived hearts, smoking in your early years, and becoming fatter than any generation before has left you with lots of crusty cells. The debris within your tissue has been there for years. If you are overweight, this debris has been around for as long as those extra pounds have been insulating you. PLUS ten years.

Brain autopsies tell the tale.

Proteins build up in a damaged brain. This damaged brain leads to Parkinson's, Alzheimer's disease and dementia. The beginning of these problems don't start with your genetics; they start with inflammation.

After ten year of constant inflammation, your gray matter's genetics can trigger all sorts of brain diseases. The chemistry produced by the combination of fasting and high ketones reverses the inflammatory grime afflicting most Baby Boomers' brains. In fact, this chemistry decreases the swelling of the brain. Fasting and high ketones trigger your cells to start eating the 'junk' that has been messing up your brain's electrical signals and activity for years.

Brains destined for dementia have been squirreling away extra proteins for years before you experience your first memory glitch. If you could take a virtual tour around your brain the year before your memory starts to go, you would see lots of these crusty, extra proteins also known as plaques or neurofibril tangles.

Already experiencing memory problems? Start eating up plaque! Stimulate autophagy by adopting a keto lifestyle with fasting.

Hopefully, I have your attention! That strange word with a comical definition should interest every Baby Boomer.

How do you switch on your personal autophagy processes? Thankfully, Nobel laureate Ohsumi's research sheds light on this science. Autophagy is a very regulated process where your cells break down components and then use those parts as nutrition.

Our cells are programmed to die. When will your cells die?
That depends on how well you've taken care of them.

Apoptosis (pre-programmed death) is triggered when cells get old and worn down. Different cells in the body live longer than others, but they all have an end date-a predestined date that they will die. That date comes quicker if they are poorly built or constantly inflamed.

A similar process happens on the subcellular level. Instead of throwing out the whole cell via apoptosis, autophagy replaces just a section of the cell. This process doesn't kill the whole cell.

APOPTOSIS says, "This cell is crap. Time is up. Throw it all away."

AUTOPHAGY says, "This section of the cell is crap. Let's break it down and use it as fuel for the rest of the cell."

Autophagy describes your cells' internal housekeeping processes. Your cells vacuum up debris and recycle these parts as fuel. Cells clean up the old worn out or defective proteins inside them and toss them into the furnace, the mitochondria. Thankfully, those burning flames of the mitochondria are right there inside the cell too.

Why should you care?

Answers: Flabby skin after weight loss.

It is embarrassing to share how many Boomer patients have said these words to me, "Doc, I don't want to lose that weight. It will leave me with too many wrinkles."

I just have shake my head while typing that.

I've got some great news for you. If you lose weight while stimulating autophagy, your body will 'eat' those deformed skin cells that caused your wrinkles. You will 'eat' those extra blood vessels, fat cells, and connecting cells as you lose weight. Without that left-over, unneeded tissue, your skin connects tightly to the overlying tissue. This results in tight, toned skin. No batty arm wings for you!

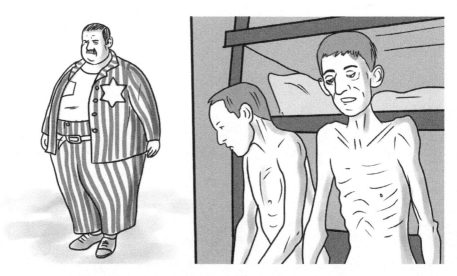

Take a trip through history. Lookup Holocaust victims in World War II concentration camps. The photos of these people show tight skin and no flabby or wavy folds of skin.

Some were overweight when they entered those camps. Sadly, they lost lots of weight during their months or even years of imprisonment. These individuals were in a state of ketosis and fasting for most, if not all, of their confinement.

A Tale of Two People who Lost 100 Pounds:

One loses 100 pounds while stimulating autophagy. The other woman used a low-calorie torture diet to lose the same amount of weight. No autophagy involved.

The autophagy patient's body successfully absorbed all of her flabby skin cells and use the cellular parts as fuel. Additionally, there is no extra flesh in her arms, butt, or abdomen. Her body used that protein- and fat-filled tissue to feed her system during her fasting period. She saved herself the pain and expense of having to go under a plastic surgeon's knife just to cut those 'wings' of flab off.

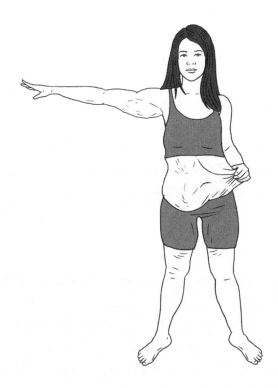

In the medical field, these leftover tissues are collectively called a 'curtain of skin.' Removing all this excess tissue by way of surgery carries a huge risk of blood loss. Until I saw this with my own eyes, I underestimated how many blood vessels remained in that tissue after tremendous weight loss.

The restricted-calorie patient also lost weight and got skinnier. No doubt about that. But her weight loss program left behind thousands of blood vessels, connective tissue cells, skin cells, fat cells and more.

Patients who choose to cut that curtain of skin off after their weight loss suffer from large rope-like scars where the surgeon connected the remaining skin back together. They are not soft and flexible scars-they are keloid roadmaps.

Why?

One word: INFLAMMATION.

Nothing says inflammation like blood when it is outside of your blood vessels. Thousands and thousands of little threads of blood vessels remain in that curtain of skin. Without the help of autophagy, there is no process to remove the leftover blood vessels and tissues that used to hold, feed and support those layers of fat. Regardless of how skilled your plastic surgeon may be, shutting down every tiny blood vessel before stitching the edges of the skin closed leaves some gnarly-looking scars.

The imagery unsettles me and my patients as I tell them of their options. However, it is inspiring to see folks lose 100 pounds and NOT have this 'flabby arm-wings' problem. People do manage to lose weight and avoid flabby skin-only if they trigger the process called autophagy. By activating the body to recycle the energy found in the excess protein and fat tissue of flabby skin, the human body can literally eat itself into a tighter, firmer, and better-looking form.

How do you trigger autophagy?

This answer involves complicated biochemistry. Thankfully, the cliff notes can be summed up in one word: FASTING.

As previously mentioned, your body chemistry during times of no eating is an enhanced version of the same chemistry you have during ketone production. By achieving ketosis before you fast, you set the stage for faster autophagy activation. Your cells can start 'recycling' their crusty parts in as little as 12 hours from the start of your fast. On the other hand, if carbs are your cells' main fuel source, autophagy kicks in several days after you stop eating.

Good news: When keto adapted you don't have to fast as long as Grandma Rose did. You don't even have to fast 24 hours. By establishing a 'fasting window' of 12 hours every day (this includes 8 hours while you sleep), you benefit from your body's recycling system. In fact, fasting daily can change the way you age.

Fasting's anti-aging benefits come directly from the autophagy triggered when people stop eating for longer blocks of time. Fasting triggers two reactions. First, to find nutrition despite the fact that you haven't eaten any calories, your body starts converting old junky proteins in your cells into energy. Second, your cells experience a burst in growth hormone production. Human growth hormone promotes muscle and bone growth. This compound also pushes your body to empty its fat cells.

As I write this chapter, I am on my fifth day of fasting. My average blood sugars hover in the 50-80s and my ketones have steadily risen to the 4.0-5.5 range. Because this fast occurred after months of ketosis, the transition was not difficult. In fact, I would agree with the literature that the first two days are the hardest. After that, each day seems to produce a higher level of energy and clearer thinking. Two of my patients in their 80s have recently adopted a pattern of seven days of fasting followed by seven days of ketosis feasting. This pattern of eating was selected to give them the best chances of autophagy in their remaining years.

How do you stop autophagy?

Just start eating again. When your body gets glucose from your food, insulin production is triggered and this hormone slams the brakes on autophagy. Even the smallest amount of insulin can stop 'energy recycling' in its tracks. Autophagy is only possible through fasting. A ketogenic diet allows you to slide back into a fasting state much easier and faster compared to multiple days needed with a carb-heavy diet.

BOOMERS: EAT YOURSELF!

Chapter 23

Lessons from Dr. Bosworth:

GASTRIC BYPASS: ALL GUTS, NO GLORY

Gastric bypass is probably one of the greatest crimes committed against Baby Boomers in medical history. It is an atrocious approach to weight loss. Clinicians who recommend it ignore the body's weight loss chemistry. Even worse, once the surgery was over patients were abandoned. The typical surgical package includes a year of follow-up. Once those 365 days are over, the surgical team disappears. Patients are left with their new rerouted anatomy and serious nutrient malabsorption problems. Patients are completely on their own as they attempt to manage the medical consequences of bypass surgery. On. Their. Own.

These obese patients entered surgery with 'inflamed brains' from years of high insulin and no ketones. They underwent a major surgery. No matter what label the surgery team used, mini-bariatric or sleeve bypass or gastric banding, there's no denying this type of surgery is major. This procedure added more inflammation and trauma to already burdened and unhealthy patients.

Next, they undergo a year of post surgery starvation. This injures their body and brain anew. With starvation-based weight loss in full swing, the year following surgery is often remembered by the patient as a cloudy, dark, and depressed time. These patients are expected to attend classes to master the advanced science behind their surgically induced, lifelong malabsorption problems. Years after this crime-of-a-surgery, patients suffer from extreme depression, a wilted immune systems, tingling or dead nerves and diarrhea with most meals.

They had no idea their gastric bypass was destroying them one day at a time. The majority of them continue to struggle with significant obesity after having spent upwards of $50,000 for this procedure.

Let me list a few of the problems found after these surgeries. The following nutrients are no longer absorbed correctly after surgery:

Thiamin, Pyridoxal Phosphate, Folate
Vitamin A, Vitamin K, Vitamin D, Vitamin B12
Omega 3 and Omega 6
Magnesium, Phosphorus, Potassium
Selenium, iodine
Zinc, Copper, Iron,

Copper and zinc levels do not return to normal causing hair loss, poor immunity, anemia and poorly functioning nerves and muscles. Surgery removed the section of their gut that's responsible for absorbing iron and many of the listed compounds above.

After surgery, these nutrients slowly decrease. Years later, gastric bypass patients live with brain fog, low energy, thinning hair, and slower disease recovery. This malnourishment is PREDICTABLE and PREVENTABLE.

If you've had gastric bypass, PLEASE follow up annually with your doctor to measure these nutrients. It is VERY IMPORTANT.

Thanks to the high-density nutrients found in keto-compliant foods, bariatric bypass patients can overcome the nutrient deficiency caused by their surgery. I insist my weight loss patients add two nutrient dense foods to their menu: liver and sardines. For real!

I show them these charts on the following page. Look carefully at the rows for sardines and liverwurst. These two food items solve a lot of deficits.

If you want your brain to operate at peak performance, you need to properly nourish it. Turn the page and use these charts to inspire your shopping list.

VITAMINS	A (IU)	B1 Thiamine	B2 Riboflavin	B3 Niacin	B5 Pantothenic Acid	B6	Folate	B12	C	D	E	K	Choline
EGGS	586	0.1	0.5	0.1	1.4	0.1	44	1.1	0	0	1	0.3	225
LARD	0	0	0	0	0	0	0	0	0	0	0	0	49.7
GRASS FED BUTTER	2499	0	0	0	0	0	3	0.2	0	0	2.3	7	18.8
HEAVY CREAM	1470	0	0.1	0	0.3	0	4	0.2	0.6	52	1.1	3.2	16.8
FETA Cheese	422	0.2	0.8	1	1	0.4	32	1.7	0	0	0.2	1.8	15.4
STEAK	0	0.1	0.1	6.7	0.7	0.7	13	1.3	0	0	0.2	0.9	65
SARDINES	108	0.1	0.2	5.2	0.6	0.2	12	8.9	0	272	2	2.6	85
LIVERWURST	13,636	0.3	1	4.3	3	0.2	30	13.5	3.5	0	0	0	0
BROCCOLI, raw	623	0.1	0.1	0.6	0.6	0.2	63	0	89	0	0.8	102	18.7

MINERALS	Calcium	Iron	Magnesium	Phosphorus	Potassium	Sodium	Zinc	Copper	Manganese	Selenium	Fluoride
EGGS	50	1.2	10	172	126	124	1.1	0	0	30	4.8
LARD	0	0	0	0	0	0	0.1	0	0	0.2	--
GRASS FED BUTTER	24	0	2	24	24	11	0.1	0	0	1	2.8
HEAVY CREAM	65	0	7	62	75	38	0.2	0	0	0.5	3
FETA Cheese	493	0.7	19	337	62	1116	3	0	0	15	--
STEAK	9	1.9	23	212	342	55	3.6	0.1	0	21	--
SARDINES	382	2.9	39	490	397	505	1.3	0.2	0.1	53	--
LIVERWURST	22	8.9	12	230	179	700	2.3	0.2	0.2	58	--
BROCCOLI, raw	47	0.7	21	66	316	33	0.4	0	0.2	2.5	--

Chapter 24
Grandma Rose: FASTING REDUX

Grandma Rose surprised everyone with her strict adherence to two servings of bone broth per day. In a flash, she arrived at the end of her second week of fasting. The oncologist visit snuck right up on us.

One hundred miles separated the oncologist's hospital from ours. He had read of her horrific turn of events from notes from her hospital stay. From her multiple scans, pages of medical notes, blood transfusion to her pooping birth canal, the grim updates set appropriate expectations. The doctor mentally processed her series of events while he factored in her age of 72 and her decade of living with cancer.

Astonishment stopped the words from leaving his throat when he opened the door to greet her. The mess of a person he had read about could not possibly match the radiant, joyful, energized woman sitting in front of him. Mary Poppins was back! At least in part.

Gathering his composure, he recalculated his words. We reviewed the situation and agreed to begin a round of much needed chemo. He reminded us that considering all the factors, we still needed a sliver of real estate in her bone marrow to grow some red blood cells, healthy white blood cells and platelets. This was mandatory to get through her crucial and life saving colon surgery.

Chemotherapy options had changed in the four years since her last treatment. This time, the doctor offered her a pill taken every day for up to a year. The good news was that we could stop the treatment if we needed. We could control the pace of the cancer-killing medication. The bad news was, the cost of the medication was over $20,000 for the first month. Wow.

In the three weeks since her abscesses started to drain, she continued to need less and less antibiotics at each turn. This repurposed use for her birth canal was a flimsy and temporary solution by any measure. The sooner we got her to a solid, stable abscess draining solution, the better she would be.

On Tuesday, twenty-three days into her fast, she took her first chemotherapy pill.

By Friday she whispered, "I think my lymph nodes are smaller."

The years I have spent bragging about her Mary-Poppins characteristics had stupefied her. Grandma Rose's positive approach, just like Mary Poppins, blinded her from reality. When she whispered her perceived reduction in those lymph nodes after only three days of medication, I was certain it was just her positive attitude talking.

Secretly, I wondered if the ketones and fasting had helped. The random times when I checked her blood ketones, she was always in the 2.0~4.0 mmol/L range. Did this steady supply of ketones weaken her cancer cells? Would this chemistry shift allow the chemotherapy to work better, stronger, or faster? I wanted to believe it.

I prayed that Grandma Rose's cancer cells would starve away from the lack of sugar in her bloodstream. I prayed that her immune system would churn out just a few perfect white blood cells to protect her. I imagined every extra drop of stagnant fluid lurking around the places it didn't belong being squeezed out.

I had daydreams about M.D. Anderson's medical team's studies that insisted on ketosis for select cancer patients.

Curiosity has been my weakness. The obsession with the idea that she could be better in such a short time did it. I hopped into my car and drove the hundred miles to the farm to see for myself. There it was. Results that surpassed all expectations.

Grandma Rose was correct. Those lymph nodes were smaller. She was right. They were. The medication had melted much of her ten-year growth-all in four days!

I could not believe what was right in front of my eyes. Bumpy marble-like masses of lymph nodes had filled her neck for so long that I forgot how slender her neck could be. The mounds of hard, dense lymph tissue in her armpits allowed my fingertips to sink into her now soft, squishy mass.

One word circled inside my mind: MIRACLE!

The hopeful feeling surging between us filled the room. It filled that old farmhouse. It saturated the whole farm.

We slept so easily that night. Peace blanketed all of us for the first time in weeks. Grandma Rose made it! She made it through. If your lymph nodes had responded that much, her bone marrow certainly had to have seen improvement. A trifecta: Her ketones rose just enough; her infections settled down just enough; her chemotherapy hit just enough. The hand of God gently rested upon us.

Every dose of chemo during that perfect storm impacted her like a month of chemo treatments had in the past. Still, one question turned in my mind. How long would it be before one of the following slipped out of balance: the ketones, her immune system, or the chemo's effect?

Reducing her cancer cell count came at a price. Grandma Rose's cancer cells died off quickly. Within days, a heavy accumulation of dead cancer cells inflamed her body. In life's long list of problems, this was not such a bad one to have. It meant the cancer was losing. But the battle ended abruptly when her system overloaded with cellular debris landing her back in the hospital. Her weakest link was infection filling guts. The insides of her bowel and those pockets of infections had all puffed up again.

OBJECTION #11: "Won't this high fat diet clog my arteries and give me a heart attack?"

The answer is NO. This is a nutritional myth that thankfully is starting to come to light. For years, we've known that high insulin levels were causing lots of troubles with cholesterol, heart disease, and brain disease. Fortunately, over the last several years, more and more experts have shown that saturated fats are not the culprit. Sticky, inflamed platelets are.

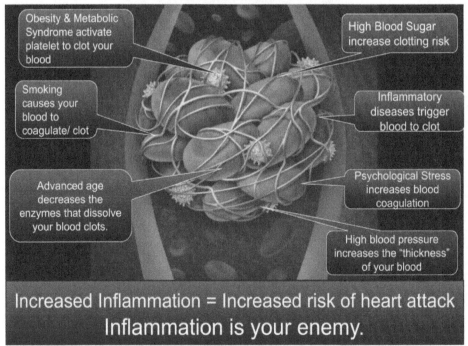

Clog Your Arteries With Inflammation
Here's what causes a heart attack.

Obesity & Metabolic Syndrome activate platelet to clot your blood

High Blood Sugar increase clotting risk

Smoking causes your blood to coagulate/ clot

Inflammatory diseases trigger blood to clot

Advanced age decreases the enzymes that dissolve your blood clots.

Psychological Stress increases blood coagulation

High blood pressure increases the "thickness" of your blood

Increased Inflammation = Increased risk of heart attack
Inflammation is your enemy.

An essential part of your circulatory system, platelets stop you from bleeding to death if you get cut. They are supposed to remain on standby until a signal tells them to plug up a leak in the system somewhere. When inflammation is high platelets get triggered to form clots. They get sticky.

High-sugar and high-carbohydrate food causes inflammation. Psychological stress, obesity and blood sugar also activate your platelets to clot by stirring up more inflammation. Small clumps of stuck together platelets, called blood clots, circulate throughout the blood vessels. These clots lodge into the tiniest of blood vessels and stop flow inside organs like the brain and heart. Other clotting triggers for platelets include smoking, diabetes, and high blood pressure. All of these make the platelets stickier and more likely to begin the clotting process.

It is a fact that there is no scientific study published linking the cholesterol you eat or the foods high in saturated fats to heart disease. They are not linked.

In the past decade, scientific research has finally concluded that there isn't a connection between consumed saturated fat and heart disease. In 2012 the British Journal of Nutrition published the findings that death from heart disease was best predicted by the percentage of calories in your diet that came from fat. The shocking results were that the GREATER your calories from fat, the LESS likely you were to die of heart disease.

Chapter 25

Lessons from Dr. Bosworth:

HOW TO GROW YOUR HGH MOTHER NATURE'S WAY

BABY BOOMERS: I am sorry. Your generation paid the highest price. At the age of 30, you were told to eat low-fat food or you'll have a heart attack.

You listened to this mantra throughout your life. Now you're in your 60s or 70s. Your fear of fat is solidly wired into your brain. 'Do not eat fat or you will die.' Oh, SNAP! I am sorry. This was the wrong advice.

I'd personally like to apologize on behalf of the medical establishment for how poorly we have advised you. You've had more surgeries than any previous generation. The medical industry talked you into over-medicating thanks to the 'packaged truths' about those drugs. We've opened your hearts, got you on *statin* meds, and stented your arteries instead of teaching you how to fix your troubles the correct way.

Instead, we should have taught you to manage your body chemistry-not re-route your blood flow. In your remaining decades, I offer you the secret to course correct your body: Growth Hormone!

One hormone can reverse every crime conventional medicine has done to you: Growth Hormone.

Human Growth Hormones' (HGH) mass media popularity started when bodybuilders injected it with the promise of mighty and lean muscles. This touchy little chemical does not work optimally when swallowed. Human Growth Hormone, or HGH, must be injected. That scares off most of my patients, but not bodybuilders. They used this hormone with great success to grow muscles. That audience consumed this drug, and soon they shared trade secrets with Hollywood and the like. Take a look at the latest movie starring a big, buff, cut actor or a sleek, lean actress. Chances are they got their physique courtesy of HGH. Attend a Broadway or Las Vegas theater show. Look carefully at the lean, strong dancers or flying acrobats. That's HGH in action.

For twenty years I've heard the desperation of patients trying to lose weight. The answer is growth hormone.

Wait. Before you rush out and shoot up with growth hormone, finish reading. This chemical compound provides a good answer for much of your middle-aged problems, but it is tricky to dose properly. Let me teach you how to get your body to produce more growth hormone. That's right, trigger your body to squirt out more growth hormone.

Endocrinologists, physicians who specialize in hormones, are thrilled about HGH. It fixes everything wrong with a middle aged, overweight, slightly depressed, low-energy person. Growth hormone reverses your age. It's THE anti-aging cure.

My medical school textbooks taught me that growth hormone decreases as you age. After age 50, your body's HGH production slows to a trickle, never to rise again.

I am here to tell you: that's not true. You absolutely can stimulate your body to make more growth hormone at any age.

Before we go into that, let's review exactly what growth hormone does.

Growth hormone. Say it out loud: growth hormone. You got it. It makes things GROW. This hormone is produced inside your brain-in your pituitary gland to be exact. Like many of the other hormones in your body, the chemical structure of growth hormone begins as a fat.

As you were developing through childhood and adolescence, this hormone told your muscles and bones to grow. Growth hormone was critical in transforming your body from a child to an adult. Naturally, the body cranked out its largest amount of growth hormone during puberty. HGH seeps out of your brain cells during sleep. Your grandma's wonderful advice to you when you were a teenager about getting lots of sleep was spot on. Well-rested teenagers produce the most robust growth hormone of all - and they produce it best while asleep. During your adolescent years, if you want the best-developed body, get deep, predictable, sound sleep.

From puberty onward, your body produces less growth hormone.

Measuring growth hormone in the human body is quite difficult. HGH only lasts for a few minutes in the bloodstream. Competitive athletes take advantage of this. They inject HGH into their systems knowing the sports doping police won't be able to measure it. Naturally, your brain squirts a burst of HGH into your body every night right after you enter a state of deep sleep. Typically, this is six hours into the sleep cycle or around 4 o'clock in the morning.

Once in your bloodstream, HGH begins a cascade of other reactions. First, your liver releases a substantial sugar dose into your bloodstream causing you to wake up. Subsequently, HGH gets to the business of what it does best, stimulating growth. It grows the following cells: immune system, skin, hair, liver, bone, nerves, muscles and many more.

To supply fuel for all this growth, HGH triggers fat cells to open up and empty their stored energy. In comparison, this is the opposite of what insulin does to those same fat cells. In the presence of growth hormone, your storage cells release fat into your bloodstream. HGH improves your overall energy levels by freeing up stored fuel. It revs up your metabolism, brightens your mood, and suppresses your appetite. It also boosts your sex drive! What a great drug, right?!

Conversely, low HGH causes fatigue, decreased stamina, depressed mood, decreased muscle mass and strength, thin and dry skin, increased fatty growth, slow thinking, and decreased bone density.

Can you see why this hormone is perfect for every middle-aged person looking to reverse the effects of aging?

At this point, you're probably asking, why don't people just shoot up HGH?

HOLD ON. Don't do that.

Hijacking the squirt gun for HGH has some SERIOUS consequences. Those experts I mentioned earlier called Endocrinologist - they
know what they are doing. These super smart, specialized doctors have
tried many ways to get the HGH formula exactly right. When they overshoot and inject too much hormone, bad things happen.

Overshoot and you will soon become a moody, pimply diabetic
with high blood pressure and an enlarged heart. Not to mention, men start
growing boobies. That is not a joke. That's real. Their breasts go from
boy breasts to milk-producing girl breasts due to the excess HGH converting to estrogen. That extra estrogen also shrinks their testicles.

When HGH dosing is not correctly calculated and timed, the effects can be gnarly. Although teenagers depend upon growth hormone to
lengthen their bones, the adult bones are fused and can't grow any longer.
However, too much HGH in an adult morphs their face bones into a Ne-
anderthal-like look. Overshoot that HGH and their forehead thickens and
their jaw bones overgrow. Additionally, a poorly timed injection of HGH
into adults will cause mood swings and pimples that flash you back to
your teenage years. Too much HGH at the wrong time and you can take a
perfectly decent Dr. Jekyll and awaken the evil Mr Hyde.

Also, injecting HGH for unapproved purposes is illegal and expensive.

Mother Nature Does A Brilliant Job

It turns out nature does a way better job squirting the perfect dose at the right time to give you all of the awesome benefits without breaking the law, draining your wallet and accidentally morphing you into a raging monster.

How do we get more of this fantastic hormone that melts your fat away, increases the strength of your muscles, concentrates the density of your bones, boosts your energy, erases your wrinkles, focuses your brain, improves your memory and sparks your libido the 100% safe and natural way?

Answer: FASTING.

Take a deep breath. It's not the end of the world. Fasting isn't your enemy.

Granted, I don't bring this up to patients until they have been in nutritional ketosis every day for at least SEVERAL weeks. Sometimes, we wait months. If a patient tells me how little they feel hungry, I might ask that patient to fast sooner. This advanced education about growth hormone and fasting promises many benefits. If I broach this subject too early in patients' education, they do not believe me.

"I know you told me this, doc, but I didn't believe you. I just don't have the hunger I used to."

Remember, hunger is caused by your blood glucose fluctuations. You feel less hungry when your glucose level remain stable thanks to ketosis. Entering the second or third week of ketone production, patients find they unintentionally skipped a meal for the first time in their life.

Telling patients about this before they experience it has not been rewarding. They thought that was impossible.

When in your third week of ketone production, I encourage you to try to eat one meal a day for two days. Have a nice, high-fat-low-carb supper. Eat until you are full. No snacking after supper. Go to bed if you feel like eating. When you get up the next morning, have black coffee without food. Pick a busy day to do this. Allowing your mind to be distracted from food is one of the keys to success. If anyone offers you food, say these words, "No thank you. I am fasting today. Please, don't tempt me." Seriously. Practice saying those words out loud. They work like a charm.

Drink water or coffee. Put a few Pink Himalayan salt crystals in your pocket for easy access. If you experience a wave of hunger, put one of those salt crystals on the tip of your tongue.

Then pause.

Listen. Listen for the shift in what that salt crystal does to your system during a fast. Take that moment to honestly assess what happens. I have learned so much about my own coping skills in this tiny, reflective, mindful moment.

Most often you can get past waves of hunger and get to supper without eating any calories.

This sounds crazy when you have not experienced it before. For years, this was an impossible task. So impossible, I could not imagine it. A body fueled on glucose does NOT miss a meal. You get shaky, you can't think or stay focused, and food becomes an obsession.

When your body is fueled by fat, hunger pangs and cravings disappear. As long as you stay hydrated, you can easily go 24 hours between meals. If the body needs fuel, you are minutes away from producing ketones from your stored fat. Your insulin stays low enough to allow your body to release and convert energy as it needs.

If you need to lose weight, you have lots of stored energy you can tap. The previous weeks of producing ketones set up your body chemistry to produce and access fat-based fuel.

Let's get back to the typical Baby Boomer. You find yourself in your mid-50s, 60s, or 70s. You've got that extra flab. How can you empty those fat cells?

GROWTH HORMONE

Not the illegal, expensive injectable kind of HGH. Your body will not forgive you when you overshoot that hormone. This compound is just too easy to mishandle. There's a better, safer, cheaper, smarter and easier way. No needles required. Start with three weeks of peeing ketones. No cheating. You must begin with three weeks of ketosis. Then migrate to the goal of eating one meal a day. Unleash the power of the anti-aging effect of HGH. Each surge of hormone at 4 AM will build upon yesterday's results.

One more drop from key cells in your brain each morning will transform your body. No, you won't be turned into a Neanderthal. Instead, HGH will reverse your body's clock. Best of all, your body determines what the proper dose is. There's no chance of overshooting this sensitive biochemical.

The net effect? In one year, you can achieve the following: less wrinkles, clearer thinking, longer focus, improved libido, thicker skin, denser bones, and higher energy. You get all these benefits on top of HGH emptying your fat cells and growing muscle mass. Remember it is a GROWTH hormone. Boomers, this is your hormone! Start making it now.

Intermittent fasting with only one meal per day for one whole year, increases your HGH production. If that's too extreme for you, fast intermittently for 4 of the 7 days of each week. That's one meal a day for four of seven days.

There are many social and psychological shifts patients must do before they can fast successfully. When you have conquered the fear of only eating once a day, you will unleash options you did not know were available.

Once my patients have fasted successfully by eating only one meal every 24 hours for several weeks, I then introduce them to longer fasting periods.

Before you dismiss this as downright loony, take a look at this study from 1982. Look at the HGH chart of the participants. They start off with a minuscule amount of HGH at 0.73ng/ml.

Now look at their numbers as they fasted day after day. By the end of the 36 days of fasting they have increased their HGH by six times. WOW! All without the side effects and cost from injections.

Kerndt PR et al. Fasting: The History, Pathophysiology and Complication. West J Med 1982 Nov; 137:379-399

TABLE 3.—*Serum Glucose, Insulin, Glucagon, Growth Hormone, Total Lipids and Triglyceride Levels in Our Subject Before, During and After Fasting*

Day of Study	Glucose (mg/dl)	Insulin (μIU/ml)	Glucagon (pg/ml)	Growth Hormone (ng/ml)	Total Lipids (mg/dl)	Triglyc-erides (mg/dl)
Prefast Period						
Days Fasting	96	13.5	138.7	0.73	530	72
Fasting Period						
5	63	2.91	222.1	2.92	430	118
12	74	5.31	161.8	4.10	440	122
19	71	2.64	248.5	7.95	410	136
26	77	1.50	327.8	9.86	400	101
33	76	1.34	727.8	3.12	470	111
36	56	2.55	198.2	4.51	400	124

This study showed the increase of HGH as patients fasted for over a month. Hormones of keto adapted patients show benefits with fasts as short as 24 hours.

Please don't let this example of extended fasting intimidate you. It is meant to show you the potential hidden within your body. Start with consuming only 20 grams of carbohydrates or less. Many of my patients feel so much better with ketosis, that we never need to advance the conversation to fasting. Like any of life's changes, start with a step and stay at that step until you master it. Then take the next step.

Chapter 26

Grandma Rose: PAIN & SUFFERING

Twenty-eight days of fasting. The final five of those days delivered Grandma Rose's chemotherapy. On that twenty-eighth day of fasting Grandpa rushed her back to the hospital.

We didn't want to admit it but surgery was the unspoken and unwelcome option that hung in the room.

Two weeks of intense medical care filled Grandma Rose's calendar before that scalpel sliced open her abdomen to remove her perforated, infected bowel.

In the end she received only 7 of her 365 chemotherapy doses prescribed. Grandma Rose's battle score versus CLL before those seven doses was GR:1 CLL: 150,000

After chemo treatment, something wondrous happened. Maybe it was this amazing new medication. Maybe ketosis robbed her cancer cells of their needed glucose. Maybe it was both.

The facts remained the same: seven doses of chemotherapy melted her cancer so quickly, that the debris from all the dead cells became our new enemy.

Those dead cells inside Grandma Rose's body sparked a frenzied process to remove them. Her body hardly noticed the removal when she gradually lost a few dead cells every day. When a large number of cells died all at once, the removal process threatened to overwhelm her system. Her body's microscopic clean up crew was equipped to handle only a few dead cells daily. It could rally and mop up a big mess now and then. Cleaning up the aftermath of a massive cancer cell die off was another thing entirely. How did her body respond to this? It swelled up. Inflammation.

Grandma Rose had so much expansion in her pelvis that her intestine swelled shut and stopped altogether. The infected abscesses and diverticula flared up first, and then spread. The chain of cancerous lymph nodes running down her spine passed their engorged toxicity to every organ in her pelvis.

The CT scan showed so much inflamed tissue that we could not see where one organ ended, and the next one began. Her doctors put her on complete 'bowel rest.'

In many ways, this was no different from what she was doing at home, except for one thing. Using standard medical care, the medical team hydrated and nourished Grandma Rose through the standard infusion of sugar water. Yes. Now sugar infused directly into her veins.

Remember how I shared that each sugar or glucose molecule holds onto about 100 molecules of water? Do you recall how the drop in someone's blood sugar when they first go into ketosis removes a whole bunch of water? Well, Grandma Rose had the reverse of this. Her ketone-adapted system had evacuated all extra water molecules by keeping her ketones high and her blood sugars low. One droplet at a time, the infusion reversed all of that. Along with that sugar came gallons of extra water.

By the third day of sugar infusions, her whole body was swollen. Her legs, her abdomen, her face. Her eyes were swollen shut. Everything! Millions of glucose molecules held onto every water droplet in her body-nearly swelling her to death. Thanks to inflammation she gained 30 pounds in three days.

The antidote to her extra fluid was strong diuretic medication pulling water out of her kidneys. Little by little urine dripped into her bag. The balance of all that misplaced water tipped the scale back towards normal. The situation improved just enough to allow surgery.

Once in the operating room, the surgeon found sticky inflammation everywhere in the bottom of her abdomen. Strings of gooey tissue seemed to have grown out of nowhere. The web of dense, slime wrapped around every part of her lower pelvis. The mass refused to separate without tearing. One choice remained. Her surgeon traced her bowel hose upstream until he found a section that was not swollen. He re-route the healthy section of her bowel to the outside of the abdomen through a colostomy opening.

Seven more calendar days passed before we saw Grandma Rose's cheek bones again. Stopping her intravenous sugar happened on day four. Her swelling faded quickly after she started producing ketones again.

In one hospital stay Grandma Rose said GOOD-BYE to:
- a section of her colon
- uncontrollable tummy pain

- bowel movements
- farting
- lots of cancerous white blood cells and
- thirty pounds of extra fluid

She also said HELLO to:
- a fancy new scar down the center of her tummy
- a colostomy bag
- the bathroom floor when she fell one night
- a ton of sleep, and
- steady improvement walking, eating and caring for her 'new' self.

She juggled a drainage tube coming out of her abdominal cavity, a PICC line out of her left bicep, a bladder catheter, a bunch of bandages, and steady stream of bloody discharge from her previously pooping vagina.

Despite all that, Grandma Rose held Mary Poppins' straight, dignified posture as she slipped into my passenger seat. We headed home.

As the hospital faded in my rear view mirror, we cautiously drove away. Each bump or slight pull of the car arrested our breathing. Instead of returning to the farm, Grandma Rose moved into our home.

The sound of the rising garage door triggered my sons to rush to greet us.

The night before, I held a family meeting reviewing all the ways our normal life would kill Grandma Rose. With three teenage boys in the house, our home had several potential death traps. A nasty accident threatened her from the pile of clothes on the floor, or the wrinkle in a rug, or a trash bags that slumped in the kitchen instead of going straight outside. The list seemed endless.

I thought I had most dangers covered until our epic fail on her first night at our home.

We arrived mid Sunday afternoon leaving time for a nap. Grandma Rose awoke just long enough to take her meds, change out her colostomy bag and take a few sips of broth.

During colostomy bag care, we noticed our mistake.

Somehow we left the hospital without any supplies for changing her bag.

Grandma's renowned MacGyver skills might have come in handy except her pain medication and extreme illness had dampened her problem-solving abilities. Pain meds stopped her suffering, but along with the discomfort went her sparkly, creative personality.

We headed to bed with plans to go to the supply store right after her 8AM doctor's appointment on Monday morning. .

Thankful for a quiet and restful night, we anxiously peaked at her bag the next morning. We shared a silent stare at the brimming colostomy bag stuck to her tummy. It was going to be close.

Thankfully the doctor was on time and by 8:45 we scooted out of the doctor's office with an expanding 'baby bump' in her shirt that looked nothing like a normal pregnancy.

We both sighed in relief as we pulled up to the medical supply store. A ray of sunlight shined onto the path as we entered.

"What do you mean there are over 2000 options for colostomy bag supplies? No, we don't have the numbers. We just have a full bag that needs to be replaced."

Two hours later, we left with one spare colostomy bag, one seal and one ring. And a promise that the other supplies will be in first thing the next morning.

The car seemed to drive itself home as Grandma Rose and I silently considered the next 24 hours. We changed dressings, emptied the current bag, rinsed it out and resealed it. We saved the spare goods in case the current system started to leak before we got supplies.

Monday afternoon and evening Grandma Rose rested and slept. She had only one episode where the pain jumped out of our control. By 8 PM we had both fallen asleep.

At 1:00AM Grandma Rose awoke to a nasty mess. The seal between her bag and the skin had popped open, and our most feared event spewed all over the night.

Grandma Rose had awoke disoriented. The warm goo on her stomach met the tight, stinging pains of her stapled skin.

Naturally, she hollered, "Help! Help!" "Annette, Help me!"

Silence.
Darkness.
Not even a stir.

She shuffled out into the hall and hollered again.

Nothing.

She called my mobile.
No answer.

Awake and determined, she waddled into the kitchen and grabbed a metal pot and spoon-and banged and banged and banged.

NADA.
Zip.
Nothing . . .

I slept through the whole thing.

The next morning I tiptoed down to wish Grandma Rose a HAPPY BIRTHDAY and found a copper pot and a metal spoon sitting on the chair in the hallway.

I peeked into her room to find her resting quietly.

Too peacefully...

I was totally unaware of her two-hour-procedure performed on herself by herself.

She had removed the dressings, took off the leaking colostomy bag, removed the adhesive-ring, and peeled off the wax seal.

She then washed, dried and prepared her skin for the next re-placement bag.

With only one spare bag, there was absolutely no space for error.

Grandma Rose handled it just like Mary Poppins. She properly measured the stoma-the part of the bowel tissue that pokes out through her skin. She pushed and massaged the wax-seal into place and put the adhesive ring over the waxed seal. She then snapped the bag on the ring, replaced the dressings, and got back to bed.

Mary Poppins never gives up.

Chapter 27

Lessons from Dr. Bosworth:

THE HARD MATH BEHIND YOUR METABOLISM

OBJECTION #12: "If you eat all that fat, you'll certainly gain weight."

Not true. Losing weight starts with changing your body chemistry. Once you become 20 or 30 pounds overweight, your body's chemistry gets locked. To reverse this, stop triggering insulin.

You burn what you eat. If you want to burn fat, you must turn on the fat-burning mechanism inside your mitochondria. If you want to lose fat, eat fat. Don't add carbs.

Focus on WHAT you eat, not how much you eat. In France the population study in 2012 showed their country as the highest in the world for the percentage of fat eaten. They topped the chart with over 40% of their calories from fat. Yet France is one of the thinnest countries in the world according to that British Journal of Nutrition.

Fat Gained/Lost = Calories In – Calories Out

This is the gospel according to Metabolism Math. According to this equation, to calculate the fat you want to lose, you must know how many calories you put into your body and subtract the calories used by your body. That is all you need to know. That's it. If you eat 1000 calories in a day and you want to lose weight, you must use more than the 1000 calories you consumed.

Clear enough, right? Unfortunately, it's wrong.

Weight loss doesn't work this way.

For over two decades, I told many patients, "Eat less. Exercise more. That's how you lose weight." My advice was wrong. This equation is flat out wrong.

Shocking, right? After all, going against that equation goes against the First Law of Thermodynamics, let alone common sense as well as conventional wisdom. But the equation is wrong.

Hear me out. Mammals are much more complicated.

Let's break this equation down.

Fat Gained or Lost = Calories In – Calories Out

Two parts of this equation are certainly measurable: 'Fat Gained/ Lost' and 'Calories In.' These two sections of the equation are easy to understand and measure.

FAT GAINED OR LOST

We can measure exactly how much body fat you have today. We can repeat that measurement several weeks from now and know precisely if you have gained or lost body fat. The best way to measure body fat is using a DEXA scan. DEXA (Dual-Energy X-ray Absorptiometry) Scan is X-ray technology used to size up lean tissue, bone density, and fat across regions of the body with amazing accuracy. Other techniques that don't use radiation include underwater weighing, whole body plethysmography, skin-fold measurements, and several other options.

My point: FAT GAINED or LOST is measurable.

CALORIES IN

We can measure 'Calories In.' Each unit of drink or food consumed has a measurement of energy. Add up all that passes your lips in twenty-four hours and you have this number. CALORIES IN is also measurable.

Fat gained = Calories In – Calories Out

CALORIES OUT

With two of the three variables measurable, we can do the math and calculate Calories Out. Right?

To double check our answer, can we measure the 'Calories Out' part of the equation? Don't nod your head so quickly.

What is the 'Calories Out' portion of the equation?

Simply, Calories Out is the total energy it takes to run your system for twenty-four hours. It represents the calories your body uses in one day to stay alive. Measuring calories out is not simple.

Calories Out includes the following five components:

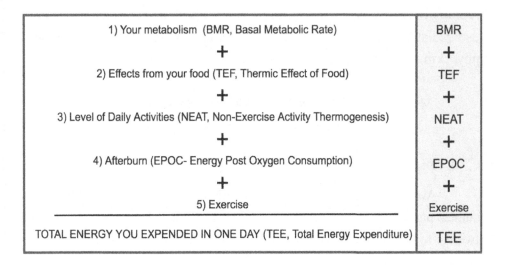

For you science geeks out there - the formula looks like this:

$$TEE = BMR + TEF + NEAT + EPOC + Exercise$$

In plain English:

Energy used to run your body = Metabolism + Energy to Process Food + Activities of the Day + Exercise + Repair from Exercise

The energy needed to run your body is much more than exercise. Let's breakdown each of these sections to get an understanding of our daily energy needs.

METABOLISM or BASAL METABOLIC RATE (BMR):

The term metabolism refers to the 'purr of your motor.' How much energy does it take to fuel the furnaces inside each of your cells? How lively are you? Would your friends describe you as a sloth or a busy bee?

Metabolism includes your breathing, maintaining your body temperature, pumping your heart, fueling your thinking, fueling your cleansing team i.e. your liver and kidneys. The list goes on for pages. Metabolism is a blanket term for a wide range of complex operations happening in your body. Also, it is not stable. It fluctuates along with your lifestyle, needs, and activities. If you think more today than you did yesterday, the equation is different. If your body had extra toxins to remove, you need a different amount of fuel.

Metabolism depends on many factors, including
- genetics
- gender (Men > Women),
- age (Young > Old),
- weight (More muscle > Less muscles),
- height (Tall > Short),
- diet (Underfeeding slows down metabolism. Pulse feeding, every 24- 36 hours, boosts metabolism.),
- body temperature (fever>normal>low body temp)
- external temperature (Hanging out in the cold requires heating the body and takes more energy than cooling it.)
- organ functions
- New Protein Production: Replacing cells in your organs.
- New Bone Production
- New Muscle Production
- Lymph System: Replacing antibodies. Fighting new invaders.
- Diseases: Is your body fighting off infection? Do you have an autoimmune disease? It takes energy to fight that.

- Brain Cognition: How much did you think today?
- Heart: How many beats pound through your heart every minute?
- Heart: How hard does your heart squeeze each beat?
- Liver: Detoxing your blood.
- Liver: Making energy. Storing energy.
- Kidney: Cleaning your blood. Making urine.
- Pancreas: Producing enzymes.
- Bowels: Moving and processing your food.
- Breathing: Lots of breaths per minute or not so much. Think of the energy needed to breath if you are suffering with asthma, or emphysema.
- Bowel Excretion: The 'slime' produced to flush, clean, and lubricate costs you energy.
- Fat Production: Storing extra calories you did not use today takes energy.
- Cancer: Cancer growing inside your system drains energy.

FOOD EFFECT or THERMIC EFFECT OF FOOD (TEF)

TEF refers to the energy used in digestion and absorption of food. Your body processes and absorbs various foods differently. For example, fats are quickly absorbed and take very little energy to metabolize. Proteins are harder to process and use up more of your resources. Foods high in fiber require the most effort to process.

Food's effect on metabolism also varies according to how much and how often you eat. Multiple small meals in a day take more energy than one large meal. The ratio of fat vs. protein vs. carbs in your meals also influences TEF.

LEVEL OF DAILY ACTIVITY or NON-EXERCISE ACTIVITY THERMOGENESIS (NEAT)

NEAT measures the energy used as you live out your day-without factoring in exercise. Sitting at this desk typing this book for over ten hours today creates a much different demand when compared to hustling around a busy medical clinic.

Did you sit for most of your day? Did you go for a walk during a break? Did you cook a couple of meals? Did you go shopping? Other than exercise, how sedentary were you?

EXERCISE

Most people get this one. In fact, usually this is the ONLY one most people think of when calculating their metabolism.

AFTER-BURN or Energy Post Oxygen Consumption (EPOC)

EPOC is the energy used to repair your body and replenish the glycogen storage that you used up during your workout or other activities. During your daily hustle, your body reached for the quick and fast energy stored in your liver. This fuel, called glycogen, is in short supply after your workout. Once your storage is used up, your body starts replenishing it. This process requires fuel.

How much energy did it take for your body to repair from your workout today? It depends on your activities as well as intensity. Did you lift weights today? Maybe it was heavier than your usual weight. Did you pull or damage your muscles during today's workout? Maybe you went for a run for the first time in years? Or did you do a two mile slow walk for your exercise?

The body does not need much energy to repair from the strolling walk. However, those muscle cells that you tore during the last back squat will need mending. That takes a lot of energy.

Imagine this. As you walk into your office, there is a sign inviting you and your coworkers to a pushup challenge. You have not done a pushup in years. The muscles needed to push your body up from the floor have been resting quietly with most of their furnaces (mitochondria) all but shut down. You decide to take the challenge and start with day one doing one pushup. Not much repair is needed. Each day you meet the daily challenge by adding a pushup to the number you did yesterday. By the end of the second week, your sore arms remind you of your new routine. Somewhere around your 14th pushup, your muscle cells said, "If this is the plan, we need to recruit some sleeping mitochondria to help out." This takes energy.

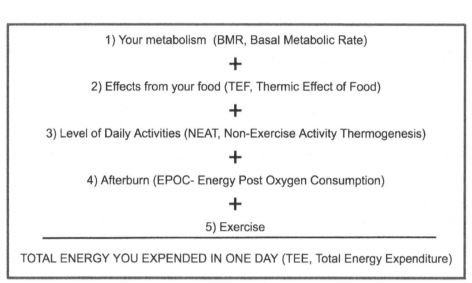

1) Your metabolism (BMR, Basal Metabolic Rate)

+

2) Effects from your food (TEF, Thermic Effect of Food)

+

3) Level of Daily Activities (NEAT, Non-Exercise Activity Thermogenesis)

+

4) Afterburn (EPOC- Energy Post Oxygen Consumption)

+

5) Exercise

TOTAL ENERGY YOU EXPENDED IN ONE DAY (TEE, Total Energy Expenditure)

Accordingly, resistance training workouts burn more energy than cardio workouts. Check your treadmill's LED display for how many calories you burned with your twenty minute fast walk. It will give you a nice number. Don't be fooled. Do pushups for one minute, then one minute of rest. Back and forth between these intervals for 20 minutes. The twenty minutes of resistance training outperforms your treadmill workout every time.

Why? Because the energy your muscles use to repair from those pushups is much greater. That's where the advantage lies.. the after-burn.

Your after-burn counts!

When trainers say "the burn the next day is not your enemy," they are correct. Your body is using up extra calories to recover.

'Calories Out' is not just exercise. All the processes below require energy to keep you alive for the day. The calories burned for the day is more than just exercise.

The number in this equation that changes the most is your metabolism, the BMR.

Eat 700 calories a day for 3 weeks, you will cut metabolism (BMR) by almost half. Then increase your calories from 700 to 1800 and it will increase by 50%.

Get cancer and you can triple your metabolism in weeks of cancer growth.

Exercise accounts for only 5 percent of the game!

Exercise never produces as much weight loss as we calculate. This is a fact. Proven again and again.

Why?

Because the human body is NOT a stable formula. We can only calculate the equation for today. But in a week, it will change. Living means adapting. We survive changes in our world because we keep up. Mammals are great at this!

Our bodies work to keep things stable. If something in your energy formula changes, another area will shift to compensate. This is called homeostasis. Our system as a whole strives to remain stable.

Not surprisingly, if we increase our daily exercise, we eat more. All the discipline in the world won't stop us from consuming more calories. Period. Several studies have proven and validate this repeatedly.

If our daily activities rise, we exercise less. This is not my opinion. Studies repeatedly show this. If you want to truly lose weight, the answer is not more exercise. Exercise is important for a number of very good reasons. It will not produce significant weight loss. It's a minor player. Emphasizing exercise detracts from the real issue of dietary problems. When one thing changes, something else in the system counters that change. We compensate. We adapt.

If you want your energy to rise, change your fuel. The easiest way to boost your metabolism is to switch fuels. Fuel your body on sugar and your furnaces put out 2 units of energy for every glucose molecule burned.

Burn fat and 32 units of energy are produced for every single ketone. This is not just a math equation for losing weight. The increased production from ketones raises your metabolism along with your thinking, focus, energy and repair rate.

Chapter 28

Grandma Rose: MEET SQUIRT

Three weeks after Grandma Rose's colostomy, we named her intestinal opening-a.k.a. her stoma-Squirt. Little did we know that such a seemingly small opening requires so much work and attention. Despite our best efforts, there is an ever present threat of Squirt leaking, not to mention 'burping' to relieve excess gas. The bag can last several days, but to prevent skin irritation, the whole assembly must be changed. This takes about an hour if everything goes right. Up until this point, each challenge seemed manageable as we learned to figure out one obstacle after the next.

The day we named Squirt, Grandpa visited his sweet wife. Before she could move back to the isolated sanctuary of the farm, both Grandma and Grandpa needed to get up to speed on caring for Squirt.

We taught him all about the importance of measuring the diameter of Squirt, pulling off the old adhesive without tearing skin, gently cleaning her mending scar, packing the spots that have yet to close, and then-the toughest part-getting rid of the wax.

Squirt needed to be caulked with a ring of wax. With each change of the adhesive, the wax ring had to be molded to the size of the stoma. A couple of minutes of massaging, tugging and molding that wax resulted in the right size to fit snugly around the opening. If too much skin is visible between the edge of the wax and Squirt, skin break-down occurs.

But that day, Squirt got nervous. As soon as everything was clean and ready for wax, 'Squirt.' At first, Grandma Rose and I were startled-- looking at each other with a sideways glance. We'd never seen that before.

This was Grandpa's first day to take all this in and he could not hold back. His reaction began with the silent shaking of his shoulders, only to be followed by a full-on belly laugh. I looked away trying not to join him. Fail. The laughter caught me, and then Grandma Rose.

Returning to her prim and proper and oh-so-composed Mary Poppins' voice, Grandma Rose scolded Squirt into better behavior. "Now stop that!"

Squirt squirted again.

"That is no way to behave when we have company."
All three of us joined in the giggles.

The addition of a colostomy bag forced us to visually analyze Grandma Rose's stools. A bag collecting all waste moving through her remaining guts made it impossible to avoid. Before long Grandma Rose was able to track the timing and specifics of her stool. How much? How often? How much gas? What color? Slimy? Smelly? The list was endless.

Grandma Rose had produced ketones for over a year. She switched off ketosis for several weeks before and after her surgery. Now we were back in the saddle.

Our family had also practiced ketosis for the past year, but adding Grandma Rose as a house guest leveled us up.

She, like any colostomy patient, wanted to decrease her stool volume. Some of the vegetables puffed her bag so full of gas that she had to 'burp' it hourly. Grandma Rose preferred her daily serving of bone broth and coffee. She added one highly ketogenic meal each day in accordance with an intermittent fasting schedule.

We went to see the surgeon fifteen days after her surgery. Grandma Rose held high hopes of getting her abdominal drain out and some staples removed. After careful consideration, the surgeon said, "Nope. We can't do that yet. You're just not weaving enough of a scar to remove those staples. I'm afraid you'll split right open without them. There's still quite a nasty slime coming out of your drainage tube. We have to wait."

We left the exam room with heads bowed and shoulders slumped. The big windows and sunshine drew us into the waiting room chairs. Grandma Rose sat with Grandpa Rich. The weight of their disappointment kept them from moving. Grandma Rose was healing very slowly. Too slowly. After several silent minutes, we reflected on all the things that HAD gone right. We weren't going to let the inconvenience and discomfort of staples and drains overshadow all the blessings and improvements.

Twenty-five days passed before her surgeon finally pulled out a few staples and the drain tube. Grandma Rose continued to show signs of danger. Still, she had high ketone readings, low blood sugar levels, and a declining need for pain meds. However she logged excessive hours of sleep. She had gone from sleeping ten hours per day to nearly twenty hours daily. There was something going on inside her draining a lot of energy.

The danger sign? She was very weak and her neck was swollen.

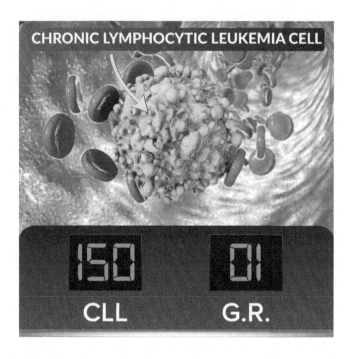

Her oncologist had bad news. Her white blood cell count had gone from an encouraging 17,000 to 143,000. Remember that with CLL, we care about doubling rates. In five short weeks, her number had sky-rocketed EIGHT TIMES. Not good.

The doctor's exam palpated hundreds of lymph nodes-no-thousands of lymph nodes. They were everywhere. They had sprung up in every nook and cranny of her body. This fresh crop of lymph nodes all shared the same size suggesting they all appeared simultaneously.

Looking back, the day she left the hospital her CT scan revealed the reason why Grandma Rose was fatigued and healing too slowly. There they were. All ten thousand of them. Staring at me like baby gremlins in the night just waiting to take over. Not one of us had noticed them.

We had all missed it. Her budding new lymph nodes were filled with cancer. This looming threat hid in the bogginess and swelling. Her CLL outsmarted us yet again. My head swam in a fog of disappointment, surprise and helplessness.

We were too focused on her surgical complications, infections, extra fluid, possible pneumonia, clogged drainage tubes, oozing staples, and a colostomy bag- minus her replacement supplies. All the while CLL had a nasty surprise for us. I told myself that even if we had seen those budding lymph nodes, we could not have done anything. She was just too sick for one more thing.

Thousands of lymph nodes filled her CT scan. I sat staring at the images wondering how to tell her.

In twenty five days, these little monsters went from hidden larvae to palpable, full grown cockroaches. We felt them budding under her skin.

We needed to destroy these cancer nests.

The oncologist started her back on chemo.

This specific chemotherapy medicine had been the same chemical that melted her cancer from 150,000 to 17,000. Last time around, she only tolerated seven of the 365 doses prescribed. After a few doses, her body suffered an intense inflammatory response which led to her needing a colostomy bag.

I can't help but suspect that we unwittingly fed those cancer cells. Sugar dripped into her bloodstream through hospital dextrose tubes. Grandma Rose received a sum total of three weeks of dripping poison.

Had I failed? Was my decision to keep this all a secret wrong? Should I have bulldozed my way through, forcing the doctors to keep her sugar-free? Had my decision to avoid hospital drama put her in greater danger? Would I pay the ultimate price for my failed courage?

Tears streamed down my face as I remembered her eyes' grotesque puffiness three days after surgery.

I imagined the disruption I would have caused had I challenged the standard sugar treatment in that moment. That conflict would have caused harm too.

If God granted me a replay of those six weeks, which outcome would have been better?

I will never know for sure.

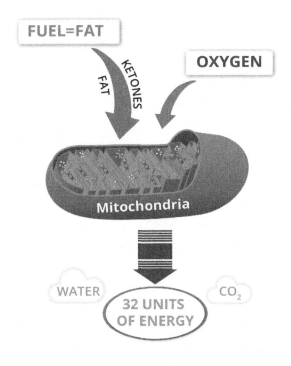

FUEL=FAT

FAT

KETONES

OXYGEN

Mitochondria

WATER

CO_2

32 UNITS
OF ENERGY

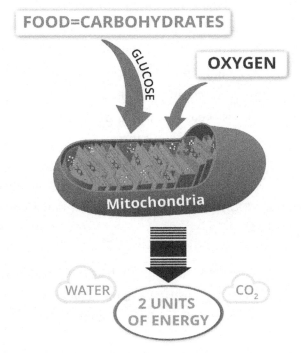

FOOD=CARBOHYDRATES

GLUCOSE

OXYGEN

Mitochondria

WATER

CO_2

2 UNITS
OF ENERGY

Chapter 29

Lessons from Dr. Bosworth:

THE SCIENCE BEHIND MCT SUPPLEMENTS

If this is the first keto book you have ever picked up, you may not have heard of these three magical letters: MCT. If you are seasoned keto veteran, you still ought to read this section with a high level of focus. MCT stands for Medium Chain Triglycerides. Let's get to the truth about them. MCT supplements are powders made from the types of fats that your body converts into ketones. Due to their purity, taking MCT supplements boost ketone levels quickly and efficiently. Watch out. There is a lot of misinformation out there.

Triglycerides are fats floating in your blood. Every time you see the word *triglyceride*, think of the fat that I could see if I drew some of your blood.

These fats are sorted based on the length of their molecular chains. Short triglyceride chains have 4-6 links each. Long chain fats have 12 or more links. Medium chain triglycerides, MCTs, have 8 to 10 links of fat. Much like Goldilocks, MCTs are not too short, not too long-they are just right. They are 'medium.' Just the right size.

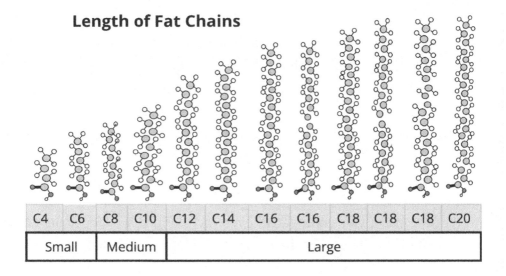

Length of Fat Chains

C4	C6	C8	C10	C12	C14	C16	C16	C18	C18	C18	C20
Small		Medium		Large							

Just the right size for what? Just right for slipping through a special nutrient trap door hidden in the first part of your small intestine. This trapdoor is your portal vein. It allows direct and almost instant absorption of certain select nutrients. Normally, your body absorbs food through its gut lining. Nutrients then enter your lymph system, a filtering safety net. They trickle through-getting sorted, screened, and shuffled before filtering into your bloodstream. For your survival, this slower lymph network protects against the entrance of any toxins, poisons, or bacteria.

Special valuable foods gain direct entry to your blood through the portal vein-that trapdoor. These select foods bypass all the sorting and shuffling happening in your lymph system. This is a risky way to allow nutrients into your body. The value of that morsel must be high enough to be worth the risk. If your body messes up and allows a toxin to enter through this back channel, you won't remain alive for long.

After entering into the portal vein, the next stop for that VIP morsel is your liver located centimeters away. Your liver converts all these fats into ketones.

MCTs are one category of nutrients allowed through this special entrance. In fact, all fats with 10 links in their chains or shorter fit through the trapdoor and are rapidly converted into usable ketones. All other fats use the standard absorption process trickling through your lymph system for 2-3 hours before entering your circulation. For the VIP fats that fit through the trap door, your liver rapidly turns them into ketone energy your body can use immediately.

As a baby, you stored fat all over your body. If we biopsy the fat in the layers swaddling a healthy baby we find high amounts of fat with 8 links of fat, called C8, as well as high amounts of fats with 10 links in each chain, called C10. Infants fill their cells with this high energy fat. How come? Speed. C8 and C10 quickly convert into abundant ketone fuel. Between milk feedings, a baby efficiently taps this fat storage system for quick energy. This is an evolutionary advantage. When food is scarce, babies survive by fueling from their stored fat. A fast growing baby requires quick access to an abundant energy source it can convert rapidly.

Why should you care about any of this? Some of you won't care. You will transition to a high fat, ketogenic diet and eventually your system will purr along on a ketone fueled motor. I wish I could say that from here on out you will live happily ever after.

Most of you, unfortunately, won't enjoy such a perfect journey. Your first attempt at keto will be new and interesting. Ketosis happens and you feel better. Weeks later, your carb intake sneaks back up and your ketones fall. Ketosis' benefits fade and you bounce out of the keto wagon completely. Your newfound keto lifestyle did not become a life-long habit.

Your initial ketosis success fades further and further into memory. You felt better when you did it and you'd like to try again but hate the suffering of keto transition. Many people have a rough time with the mood and energy slump they experience between giving up carbs and ketosis.

People switching to a keto lifestyle use MCT supplements as a shortcut to the transition. They buy these products to avoid the side effects found in the slump when your body goes from glucose to ketones. The package labels for MCT supplements promise rapid ketones and therefore lower side effects. Pay Attention! The only fats that produce rapid delivery of ketones are 10 links or shorter. They must fit through your trapdoor to deliver on that promise.

C8 fits. C8 is the chemistry shorthand for triglyceride compounds with 8 fat chain links. This is called caprylic fatty acid. C6 is termed caproic. C6 fits through the trapdoor and is a short chain fat. C10, capric, also fits. Nothing else will work. C12 is too long. These longer fatty chains trickle through your lymph system just like the fat found in butter and heavy whipping cream. These longer chain fats may convert into ketones, but they take more time to process.

Pricey supplements sell you on the speed of their ketone formulation. It is easy to get fooled into paying for fats that are too long. These do NOT metabolize quickly.

For example let's look at coconuts. Advertising teams linked the letters MCT to coconuts. Coconut fat is made up of 85% long triglycerides-too big to squeeze into your portal vein. Slick marketers focused on the 15% of coconut oil that does fit. They convert coconut oil into powder form and market it as MCT. Look closely at this chart to see the size of different fats. Notice the three smallest fats found in coconuts are called similar names: caproic, caprylic and capric. With chains 6, 8 and 10 links long, they all fit into your portal vein and turn into ketones rapidly.

Length of Fat Chain		Name	Type of Fat	% Found in Coconut Oil	Molecular Structure
Small Chains	C4	Butyric	Saturated	None	
	C6	Caproic	Saturated	0.5%	
Medium Chains	C8	Caprylic	Saturated	7.8%	
	C10	Capric	Saturated	6.7%	
Long Chains	C12	Lauric	Saturated	47.5%	
	C14	Myristic	Saturated	18.1%	
	C16	Palmitic	Saturated	8.8%	
	C16	Palmitoleic	*MUFA	None	
	C18	Stearic	Saturated	2.6%	
	C18	Oleic	*MUFA	6.2%	
	C18	Linoleic	**PUFA	1.6%	
	C20	Arachidic	Saturated	0.1%	

*MUFA: MonoUnsaturated Fatty Acids   ****PUFA:** PolyUnsaturated Fatty Acids

These three fats come from the same root word: *caprine*. Caprine refers to goats. These fats are found in high amounts in goat products. If the goat industry hired a better marketing team, goats would be associated with MCT instead of coconuts.

The CLINCHER: MCT OIL POWDERS are not created equal. Use MCT C8:C10 powder to boost your ketone production. Don't waste your money on fats that are too long. Read the ingredients label. If the MCT's root word is not *caprine* it is the wrong size to be a rapid converter. Longer fats take hours to process through your slower, safer lymph system arriving in your circulation at the same time as the rest of your food. If you want C12, it's cheaper to use a scoop of coconut oil.

For fast ketone production, use MCT C8:C10.

Chapter 30

Grandma Rose:

THE EVIL EMPIRE STRIKES BACK

Back to the numbers game. After the oncologist stared at the startling 143,000 CLL lab report, he struggled with the disbelief that it could rise so quickly. A repeat test came back at 145,000 a few days later burying our hope of a mistake. The fatigue, fullness in her neck, mounded masses in her armpits and growths in her groin were all oversized lymph nodes. These findings validated her soaring numbers. The cancer was back and growing fast.

The oncologist restarted her chemotherapy and ordered a recheck after 7 doses. The last time she took this medication, a few pills caused an inflammation explosion. This time, her cancer doubling rate was so high that we were thankful for the close follow up.

Before Grandma Rose headed back to the farm, we reviewed our keto plan. In the preceding weeks, she thought she stuck closely to it. She drew confidence from the fact that her keto urine strips turned pink every time she checked. She renewed her commitment to drink broth everyday and took my new advice to monitor her blood ketones and her blood glucose.

I advised her to step up her monitoring after reading Dr. Thomas N. Seyfried's book, Cancer as a Metabolic Disease. While his research focused on brain cancers, not chronic lymphoma, his literature was the most relevant to my mom's cancer that I could find. I instructed Grandma Rose to follow his research's advice.

His findings could be summarized as follows: Place the highest stress on the cancer cells while protecting Grandma Rose's health and vitality. Her chemo medication was going to do what it was going to do. Our goal was to create the worst environment for her cancer cells, while nourishing the rest of her body.

How exactly?

Cancer cells need sugar for energy. Lowering blood sugar to zero would destroy these cells. Sadly, that would also kill Grandma Rose, not protect her. The human body needs a minimum level of circulating glucose to survive.

The solution? Reduce her blood sugar as much as possible while flooding her system with an alternate fuel, ketones.

The higher her blood ketones, the better nourished her normal non-cancerous cells would be. I did not have the microscopic, genetic confirmation that Grandma Rose's specific cancer cells were glucose-dependent. I simply made an educated guess that they were. I based my guess on a few clues from her history. During her first six weeks of ketosis, her CLL score dropped substantially-thirty percent! Recall that she had pushed off taking chemotherapy for nearly two years at that point. Her results exceeded my hopes.

My confidence that her cancer lived off glucose grew when I saw how fasting helped her through many challenges. She stopped eating during complications from abscesses, diverticula, and perforated bowel. These all threatened her life. Fasting seemed to help her overcome these conditions. Each time she fasted, she went from severely ill to medically stable.

During the fasts, her blood sugars were low and ketones were high. When her abscesses flared and she fasted, things strangely improved. When her bowel perforated and the doctor ordered NPO, she improved. When the surgeon removed her bowels and sugar dripped into her veins, she deteriorated and the cancer grew. Maybe I was only seeing the answers I wanted to see. Maybe I was fitting my hypothesis to her situation. One fact remained: every medical textbook said she should be dead yet she was healthier now than she had been in years.

Again, although Thomas Seyfried's research focused exclusively on brain tumors, I asked Grandma Rose to follow his protocol: decrease blood sugars as low as possible while pushing blood ketones as high as possible.

She agreed and each morning, she checked fasting sugars along with ketones. She pricked her finger and placed one drop of blood onto the glucose monitor and another drop onto the ketone monitor. She also took her daily chemo pills.

According to Seyfried's research, blood glucose should always be below 80 and lower if we could get it there. Ideally, this should be accompanied by a ketone number greater than 2.0.

To simplify these goals, Seyfried uses a ratio that divides glucose by ketones. Brain tumors showed the greatest reduction when that ratio was less than 20.

For the first 2 weeks, Grandma Rose's blood sugars ranged in the 80's and 90s while her blood ketones held strong in the 1.4 to 1.8 range. We were happy if we hit the ratio of 50. Not one time did we see ratios in the 20s.

We had two objectives to work with:
1. Raise Ketones
2. Lower Blood Sugars

Either we raise her blood ketones, or lower her blood sugars. Or both. Seyfried's brain tumor studies lowered the patient's blood sugars into the 50 and 60 range. That number unsettled me. I had never seen a healthy person with blood glucose levels that low.

I reminded myself that my clinic overflowed with people struggling with chronic disease. These were not healthy people. If a newly diagnosed diabetic came to my clinic and I instructed her to get her blood glucose down to 55-65, that advice could kill her. Diabetics' sugars often run in the 150-200 range-even with medical treatment. Their bodies and brains are steeped in toxic levels of sugar.

The human brain is the slowest ketone adaptor. A quick drop of glucose to the 80-90 range causes profound side effects. Safely dropping a diabetic's sugar level from 180 to 80 takes several weeks. Grandma Rose's glucose needed to come down by 20-30 points.

I thought about adding metformin to Grandma Rose's plan. Metformin is a prescription medication that lowers blood glucose in a safe and effective way, without pushing them too low. Adding metformin would certainly reduce her sugars. It was safe, easy and cheap. This medication might also have other anti-cancer benefits. All that was good. What stopped me from prescribing it was the risk of diarrhea. One look at her colostomy bag and I decided against it. With her surgical wound finally mended, I chose not to squeeze on Squirt just yet.

The other way to lower blood sugar in ketosis patients was to lower their daily calories. We rarely talked about calories or even measured them. Her caloric intake naturally dropped as she grew accustomed to ketosis. Obviously, when she fasted she had zero calories.

She agreed to try fasting again. We called her fasting days 'bone broth days.' Much like the time when she repurposed her birth canal, she used the salty broth to push through any hunger waves. If hunger snuck up on her, she used the power of salt to deflect those symptoms.

Fasting caused her numbers to improve. Even though she did not fast for days on end like she had done before, she had nice results with intermittent fasting. She fasted for thirty-six hours twice a week. She would eat supper on Sunday and her next meal would be Tuesday morning. Her sugars sunk into the 70-80 level and her ketones reached around 2.1-2.5. That came out to a ratio of 30-40. Although our goal was 20, we proudly celebrated of our accomplishment.

On non-fasting days, she added supplements to boost her ketone numbers. The supplements can be a little confusing. I used this chart to explain her options.

She looked at the numbers in the bottom row of that chart with eagerness. Ketones-In-A-Can offer a quick and easy ketone boost. What's not to love?

Ketones-In-A-Can are made in the chemistry lab. Unlike MCT supplements, where your liver converts ketones from special sized fats, these ketones are ready made. Indeed, one scoop and her blood ketones shot into the 3.0-3.8 range. She quickly learned their downside. Chemists make Ketones-In-A-Can by connecting minerals such as potassium, sodium, magnesium or calcium to synthetic ketone molecules. If the chemist uses too much magnesium or potassium in the concoction, YUCK!

Also, these salts pull water into the bowel. When Grandma Rose drank too many Ketones-In-A-Can she turned her colostomy bag into a squirt gun. Squirt stayed mad for 2 days with diarrhea.

Typically scientists use the antidote of sugar to something that tastes that rotten. But not in the ketone lab. Instead, chemists add different artificial sweeteners. These also cause loose stools.

The additional sugar substitutes found in Ketones-In-A-Can triggered Grandma Rose's pancreas to produce insulin. Even though these substitutes don't have the chemical structure of sugar, their sweetness tricked her brain to think they are the real deal. Accordingly her body released insulin and craved more sweet flavors the rest of the day. Insulin STOPPED her ketosis, and this sent her blood sugars into a cycle of falling and rising. Insulin pushed sugars into her cells and out of her blood. Grandma Rose did not feel good when her sugars dropped that low. When she felt badly, she made poor choices.

Supplementing ketones suppressed her appetite, just like nutritional ketosis did. However, like most, Grandma Rose reported a stronger appetite suppression through fasting compared to Ketones-In-A-Can. That sounds backwards to people who have never fasted. How could your appetite go DOWN when you fast? Well, it just does. The higher your ketones go, the less you want food. The additional benefits that surge during fasting turn off your hunger. She tried a half dozen different samples before she said, "I'd rather not eat than suffer through that nastiness."

METHOD to INDUCE KETOSIS	KETONES mmol/L	BENEFITS	PITFALLS
Fasting	1-8	Rapid weight loss Autophagy	Discipline
Ketogenic Diet	1-3	Read this book.	Support System needed to stay compliant
MCT C8:C10	1-3	Uses Portal Vein to rapidly turn into ketones.	Gut rumbling from excessive MCT
Ketone Supplements (Exogenous Ketones) "Ketones-In-A-Can"	1-10	Eat your ketones. No conversion needed. Easy way to get back into ketosis after eating carbs.	Price. Taste. Diarrhea.

After that failed mess, Grandma Rose opted for MCT C8:C10. Unlike pre-made Ketones-In-A-Can, MCTs are powdered fats that your liver must turn into ketones. MCT C8:C10 had no carbs and all the right fats. A scoop of this powder quickly raised Grandma Rose's ketones for hours without a desire for food. Previously, she had mixed butter or coconut oil to her coffee instead of this powder. The fats found in the butter and coconut left her with several hours before appetite suppressing ketones arrived in circulation. MCT C8:C10 rapidly delivered only the best fats to boost her ketones.

Her blood sugars on eating days naturally ran higher than when fasting. With sugars ranging from 85-95 and ketones 3.0-3.8, her ratio spanned 22-30 that first week. Our goal was 20. We were getting pretty close. Even though she preferred fasting, it appeared that even with the all side effects, her ratio was better with the Ketones-In-A-Can.

One week after starting her chemotherapy, her follow-up exam showed no danger signs, but no big win, either. With only a smidgen of a drop in her cancer numbers, the oncologist sent Grandma Rose back home for forty more days of chemotherapy.

Week two of chemo filled Grandma Rose's shower drain with hair.

Chapter 31

Lessons from Dr. Bosworth:
DON'T READ THIS FIRST:
THE SECRET TO FAST WEIGHT LOSS

WARNING: DO NOT READ THIS SECTION FIRST. If you flipped to this page in the book wanting in on the secret of how to lose weight like a movie star, stop. You can't skip those other steps and jump straight to this advanced lesson. Seriously. This is an advanced lesson. There is a reason we used to put patients into the hospital to induce ketosis. You can hurt yourself if you don't understand the previous chapters.

WARNING: DO NOT READ THIS SECTION IF YOU ARE NOT WILLING TO COMMIT TO FOLLOW THESE RULES EXACTLY AS WRITTEN.

With all the disclaimers out of the way, welcome to the fast lane. And by fast, I am referring to weight loss.

I teach patients this lesson on weight loss when they have 'arrived.' When they get it. They have shown up at the weekly support group, they confessed all their carb sins and they want to change the course of their lives. For them, ketosis for a lifetime is not a far-fetched idea anymore. They emptied the no-nos out of their cupboards. They washed down the shelves in the pantry that used to hold bags of processed food. They pushed through that phase where adding a sugar substitute to everything seemed like a solution. They graduated from the phase where they made forty flavors of fat bombs to keep around 'just in case.' They are the real deal. Ketosis for life.

If this is you, let me help you live your healthiest life and look great, too.

You might have guessed from the past couple of lessons in this book that this involves intermittent fasting, stimulating your growth hormone, and manipulating your Metabolism Math Equation.

For this to work, you need to level up.

Step 1. Produce and Monitor Ketones for 4 Weeks

Don't try this without 4 weeks of proven ketones. If you are reading this book, you are serious about improving your health. However, you are probably not under the care of a doctor who is passionate about ketosis for life.

This rapid weight loss lesson is powerful, safe and sustainable weight loss . . . BUT YOU MUST BE KETO ADAPTED FIRST!

In cases where I did not enforce this rule, they all failed. Every stinkin' one. You must have ketones in your urine for the better part of a month for this to work. Allow me to digress.

Requiring 4 weeks of adaptation involves more than adjustments to your cell's mechanics. You must go through the process of removing temptations, cleaning out cupboards, and taking on the social challenges of becoming a ketone lover. You will be going against what society tells you. This journey is not for the faint of souls. You will be thumped over the head with the mantra that you must eat fruit. Someone will sabotage your momentum with the fear that all that fat will cause a heart attack. Others chip away at your resolve by repeatedly offering you high carb 'healthy snacks.'

If you're reading this book straight through and have never experienced high ketones with low blood sugar levels, you might think, "Doc, of course you will lose weight when you fast. But who can stick to that plan?"

You can, once you shift your chemistry. Ketosis' natural side effects will help you. Fat is your friend. Once your body's chemistry shifts to ketones, your glucose levels stabilize and gradually your hunger cycle disappears. Seriously. No matter how many patients I walk through this, my carb-addicted patients do not believe this … until the day they forget to eat. It sounds laughable, but this will happen to you.

On the Standard American Diet, your feeding signals are triggered by your blood sugars' peaks and crashes. When fueled with fat, your hunger diminishes along with your blood glucose levels. Produce ketones for 4 weeks before you try this rapid weight loss plan. That month prepares your mind, cells, and coping skills for your success.

Step 2. Buy a Blood Monitor the Week Before You Start

Proper monitoring is an essential component for rapid weight loss with ketosis. Level up by checking your BLOOD ketones as well as your blood sugars. Check them simultaneously. Originally, I bought a Precision Xtra monitor because this device measures both ketones and glucose. I randomly tested simply to satisfy my curiosity but never looked at both at the same time. When I advanced to the rapid weight loss stage of ketosis, I needed both numbers at the same time. I found it annoying coaxing my finger to bleed long enough for this set up. Each test takes only 10 seconds. However, by the time the ketone check was done, that strip pulled out and replaced with the glucose strip, my finger had stopped bleeding. I had to poke myself twice. Grrrr. When I added a separate glucose monitor and prepared both testing devices before the finger prick, it worked much better.

Supply yourself with ample testing strips. Initially you may test 3-4 times a day to gauge your progress. Monitoring centers on two valuable situations: first thing in the morning and prior to eating at the end of your fast.

Step 3. Begin Intermittent Fasting

Our goal is to boost your metabolism through intermittent fasting. Because of your keto-adaption, rapid weight loss is possible without shutting down your metabolism. Instead, your metabolism will increase.

I recommend one meal daily with at least 20 hours between meals. Since I have kids to feed, I tended to eat only at suppertime. The 20 hour minimum allowed me enough flexibility within the 24 hour cycle. These four movable hours allowed me enough adjustment that I did not have to cheat when I had to do something I could not reschedule.

Cooking while fasting is a deal-killer for me. I just can't say no. When I am doing longer fasts, the family knows because we have crockpot meals planned the whole week. I have them in the freezer and throw them into the crock pot before I leave. The meal is simple enough for the kids to help get food on the table before I screw up and eat something I am not supposed to.

A key struggle for this advanced lesson is coffee. Yep, that morning coffee has a routine so built into our lives that we talk about it first. For this advance weight loss, you cannot put fat in your coffee. Don't freak out. You are right. I told you to do that in the previous chapters. This was my main mode of survival when I first started, too. I love my coffee with heavy whipping cream in it.

However, intermittent fasting pushes your body to get its fuel primarily from your stored fat. If you're looking for your body to tap into its stored fat for its energy needs, don't ingest fat. Fast. Fast means no calories. Translation: black coffee.

Confession: I love my coffee with heavy cream. But when I started fasting, I had to skip the coffee the first few times I did this. My caffeine withdrawal headache was awful. Before long, I found a great tasting black coffee brewing process that enabled me to skip the cream. The process is called cold brew and you simply soak the ground coffee beans overnight and drip out the brew after a 12 or 24 hour soak. The taste was remarkable and not tangy or bitter. Now I fix all my coffee this way. If I want it hot, I just microwave it.

	BLOOD SUGAR	BLOOD KETONES	RATIO (GLUCOSE / KETONES)
Day 1 2:30 PM	76	0.9	84
Day 1 5:41PM	81	1.4	57
Day 2 8:18 AM	99	0.3	330
Day 2 12:34 PM	82	0.7	117
Day 2 4:48 PM	95	3.1	30
Day 3 6:09 AM	117	0.1	1170
Day 3 9:45 AM	114	0.2	570
Day 3 2:34 PM	92	0.4	230

Step 4. Measure Your Glucose/Ketone Ratio

Nothing beats real-time feedback. I insist that the patients using ketosis for rapid weight loss monitor themselves.

The first week, check your blood ketones and blood sugars 3-4 times a day. When I am following them in the clinic, I ask them to bring their numbers in for me to review. We use the same approach we used with Grandma Rose. We calculate their ketone ratio by dividing their glucose by their ketone number.

For example, look at this chart from Maurine, a 42 year old black woman with diabetes in her family. She knew that the best protection against diabetes was to achieve her ideal body weight and stay there. She had lost 30 pounds by just going keto and now wanted to remove the rest. Unfortunately, she had plateaued in her weight loss and wondered why.

She advanced to this lesson of checking ketones and glucose. At the end of three days, she returned to the clinic with these results:

On Day 3, Maurine was proud that she had reached her intermittent fasting goal of eating no calories outside of her one daily meal.

Her blood sugars and ketones did great on Day 1 and again on Day 2.

At the end of Day 2, Maurine felt amazing. She had a lot of energy and when she checked her ketones before her daily meal she found them the highest she had ever seen them, 3.1.

Take a guess at what Maurine did at the end of Day 2. She celebrated with a cup of pomegranate! Yep. Fruit is evil.

When Maurine awoke the next morning, she had NO KETONES (0.1) along with her highest blood sugar, 117. That pushed her ratio over a thousand. No weight loss that day. Talk about great feedback!

Typically the ratio needed for rapid weight loss ranges between 30-60. However, we must work with your specific metabolism. To understand your metabolism, we need the numbers. That's why you measure them: to help adapt the plan to your metabolism. In Maurine's case, she lost weight anytime she kept her ratio under 100. Maurine learned that when her ratio slipped under 100 it was a sign that her body was using her stored fat as fuel. Translation: Weight Loss.

Just like Maurine, through monitoring your glucose/ketone ratio, you will learn very quickly what is happening inside your body. The teacher is your numbers. You have to check. When your blood sugar is too high, weight loss is not possible. Your elevated sugars signal insulin to show up and fat stays locked inside your fat cells. If you skipped to this chapter and are not keto adapted, dropping your sugar without producing ketones will make you feel terrible. The science of ketosis weight loss is predictable across patients. What is NOT predictable is how YOUR system responds to food. If you are insulin resistant, a cup of carbs will kick you out of ketosis for two days. Your blood sugar will soar and your ketones will plummet. Look at that chart again. That's what happened with Maurine. Your identical twin may not be so sensitive to sugars and a few extra carbs won't block her weight loss. How do you know which one you are? Follow the science. Check those numbers to see if your choices produce the correct environment for weight loss.

Maurine fasted intermittently with one meal a day for 13 weeks and reached her target weight. The only times she stopped losing weight occurred when she stopped checking her numbers. You have to keep checking your score.

Step 5. Drink Bone Broth for Extended Fasts

Drink bone broth if you are going to fast for a period longer than 24 hours. It's warm salty liquid addresses two important factors with one solution: salt and hydration. When doing extended fasts, I take containers of frozen broth to work. On the days when I am shooting for 3, 4 or 5 days of fasting, I heat the broth up and drink the warm, salty liquid on my drive home. Works like a charm! This wonderful brew satisfies my appetite, provides nutrients beyond expectations, while salting away any waves of hunger. The family can eat while I sit at the table with them. If I skip the broth, I snitch at food and squelch my growth hormone production.

Happy Fasting!

Chapter 32

Grandma Rose: THE KNOCKOUT ROUND

By the fifth week of chemotherapy, Grandma Rose boasted that a sloth would have higher energy than she did. Strangely, fasting days were her best days for energy. On eating days while under chemotherapy, she ate one or two ketogenic meals. She reported her lowest energy when she ate. She found a tolerable Ketones-In-A-Can. One scoop per day gave her the best blood glucose/ketone ratios.

On her six-week follow up, I promised myself that I would resist the temptation to run my fingertips along her neck or stick them in her armpits. I would await the judgment of her oncologist on the size of her lymph nodes just like everyone else. We met in the lobby and the shape of her neck held my attention as she walked towards me. Five weeks had passed since I had last seen her. Her slender, lean neck captured all my attention as the rest of the world dimmed around her. My eyes slowly traced the smooth lines of her muscles sliding under her collar. Her veins and muscle contour danced across uninterrupted by any bumps from unwanted lymph nodes. Glorious. Simply glorious.

Her lab tests confirmed what I suspected. She registered a nearly 100,000 point drop in her cancer count. Upon examination, her oncologist could not find any lymph nodes. Hundreds of thousands of lymph nodes were all gone. Vanished. Removed. Six weeks of chemo and ketones left the oncologist stunned with disbelief. Struggling to trust what he was seeing, he repeated her CT scan 'just to be sure.'

This time I did not need the CT scan to know for certain how she was doing. Neither did Grandma Rose.

NOW SHE LIVES.

Every textbook predicts that Grandma Rose will die of cancer complications. So far, God has had other plans.

With the dramatic improvement in her exam and her CLL score, Grandma Rose and her oncologist agreed to stop chemo. Although her CLL score of 50,000 is not the best, given that she was 73 years old and everything else that happened to her, it was good enough for now. She eagerly said goodbye to chemo's side effects of slow healing, fatigue, and thinning hair.

For three months, she continued her ketosis with intermittent fasting as her only cancer treatment. Not only did ketones strengthen her physical body, they empowered her to fight. Instead of watching cancer take her away one month at a time, producing ketones became her torch. Ketones became her signal that represented a stronger, determined, empowered Grandma Rose.

At her follow up oncologist's appointment, her CLL score came out and our jaws dropped to the floor. Her numbers sunk further. No chemo. Only ketosis for those three months. This cancer that never drops had dropped again. Her CLL score was crushed down to 30,000.

At 73 years old, Grandma Rose's story radiates hope for many. After ten years of CLL, she was tired of the battle. Her body was old, inflamed and dying. Prepared for defeat, she surrendered. The cancer had won.

Eighteen months ago I introduced the word *ketosis* to her. Hope resurrected the day she peed her first ketone. The magic of Mary Poppins returned one mitochondria at a time. Her desire, powered by ketones, went from lifeless to a solid, steady burn.

Now she spreads hope to others living with cancer. She encourages them to, "Fight It **ANYWAY YOU CAN**! Ketosis for life!"

Chapter 33

BONUS SECTION:
7 STEPS TO STAY THE COURSE

Here are the SEVEN most important steps in sustaining your ketosis lifestyle.

1. **Connect**. Find a support group to help you through transition. This can be a formal keto group, a book club, or a couple of friends from work. Schedule a small group meeting once weekly. Make it a priority to attend meetings for at least 6 months. Changing your behavior is hard. Use relationships to ensure you stay on the wagon. Groups also help you forgive yourself when your keto transition does not pan out as you expected.

2. **Check ketones.** This single step separates this diet from every other weight loss regime. The keto lifestyle provides real-time feedback on how you are doing. Checking ketones allows you to see your progress hour by hour. Testing really takes all of the guess-work out of the process. Empower yourself by monitoring what your body is doing. Check ketones daily.

3. **Calculate your protein.** The keto diet is not a high-protein diet. Do this calculation. Find your ideal body weight in pounds. Personally, mine is 125 pounds. Convert those pounds to kilograms by dividing the number of pounds by 2.2. [125 /2.2= 57] This number (in my case 57) equals the maximum total grams of protein you should eat every day.

4. **Eat**. This is not a starvation diet. Those who skimp on their intake and eat too little sabotage their outcome. You warp your metabolism by restricting your calories before you are keto adapted. Eat until you feel full. Feeling full triggers important brain hormones which in turn stimulate your metabolism. Eat. Feel the satiety.

5. **Eat fat**. You can fuss about monounsaturated, polyunsaturated, or saturated fats. You are losing focus on the chemistry shift we want. Just focus on and eat fat.

6. **Manage your minerals**. Add salt to your liquids-especially when you begin your keto transition journey. Replace your magnesium to stop muscle cramps and improve your mood and mental processes.

7. **When in doubt eat less carbs. When in doubt eat even more fat.**

Author's Note:

Thank you for reading my book. As a first time author, I am overwhelmed with the positive feedback from readers. Thanks to you and your voice, other readers have discovered my book.

As a first time author , the most powerful gift you can give me is to share your feedback by writing a review online. I read every review posted under my book. The more FIVE STAR reviews, the more my book is suggested to other readers. Please take time to write a review. Mark it with 5-stars if you think the book deserves it. The reviews make all the difference to a first time author.

Finally, if you want to learn more about the keto diet from me connect with me at my website: www.BozMD.com

Thank you for reading my book.

Keep Calm and Keto On!!

Annette Bosworth, MD

LIMITED BIBLIOGRAPHY

1. Achanta, Lavanya B., and Caroline D. Rae. "Beta-Hydroxybutyrate in the Brain: One Molecule, Multiple Mechanisms." Neurochemical Research, vol. 42, no. 1, Aug. 2016, pp. 35–49., doi:10.1007/s11064-016-2099-2.

2. Augustin, Katrin, et al. "Mechanisms of Action for the Medium-Chain Triglyceride Ketogenic Diet in Neurological and Metabolic Disorders." The Lancet Neurology, vol. 17, no. 1, 2018, pp. 84–93., doi:10.1016/s1474-4422(17)30408-8.

3. Bergin, Ann M. "Ketogenic Diet in Established Epilepsy Indications." Oxford Medicine Online, 2016, doi:10.1093/med/9780190497996.003.0006.

4. Blackburn, Henry. "The Seven Countries Study: A Historic Adventure in Science." Lessons for Science from the Seven Countries Study, 1994, pp. 9–13., doi:10.1007/978-4-431-68269-1_2.

5. Cameron, Jameason D., et al. "Increased Meal Frequency Does Not Promote Greater Weight Loss in Subjects Who Were Prescribed an 8-Week Equi-Energetic Energy-Restricted Diet." British Journal of Nutrition, 2009, p. 1., doi:10.1017/s0007114509992984.

6. Caraballo, Roberto Horacio, et al. "Ketogenic Diet in Pediatric Patients with Refractory Focal Status Epilepticus." Epilepsy Research, vol. 108, no. 10, 2014, pp. 1912–1916., doi:10.1016/j.eplepsyres.2014.09.033.

7. Cassiday, Laura. "Big Fat Controversy: Changing Opinions about Saturated Fats." INFORM: International News on Fats, Oils, and

Related Materials, Jan. 2015, pp. 342–377., doi:10.21748/inform. 06.2015.342.

8. Castaldo, Giuseppe, et al. "Very Low-Calorie Ketogenic Diet May Allow Restoring Response to Systemic Therapy in Relapsing Plaque Psoriasis." Obesity Research & Clinical Practice, vol. 10, no. 3, 2016, pp. 348–352., doi:10.1016/j.orcp.2015.10.008.

9. Chanrai, Madhvi, et al. "Comment on âSystematic Review: Isocaloric Ketogenic Dietary Regimes for Cancer Patientsâ by Erickson Et Al." Journal of Cancer Research and Treatment, vol. 5, no. 3, 2017, pp. 86–88., doi:10.12691/jcrt-5-3-2.

10. Craig, Courtney. "Mitoprotective Dietary Approaches for Myalgic Encephalomyelitis/Chronic Fatigue Syndrome: Caloric Restriction, Fasting, and Ketogenic Diets." Medical Hypotheses, vol. 85, no. 5, 2015, pp. 690–693., doi:10.1016/j.mehy.2015.08.013.

11. D'agostino, Dominic P., et al. "Therapeutic Ketosis with Ketone Ester Delays Central Nervous System Oxygen Toxicity Seizures in Rats." American Journal of Physiology-Regulatory, Integrative and Comparative Physiology, vol. 304, no. 10, 2013, doi:10.1152/ajpregu. 00506.2012.

12. Erickson, N., et al. "Systematic Review: Isocaloric Ketogenic Dietary Regimes for Cancer Patients." Medical Oncology, vol. 34, no. 5, 2017, doi:10.1007/s12032-017-0930-5.

13. Feinman, Richard David Ph.D. . The World Turned Upside down: the Second Low-Carbohydrate Revolution. Nutrition & Metabolism Press, 2014.

14. Felig, Philip, et al. "Metabolic Response to Human Growth Hormone during Prolonged Starvation." Journal of Clinical Investigation, vol. 50, no. 2, Jan. 1971, pp. 411–421., doi:10.1172/jci106508.

15. Felton, Elizabeth A., and Mackenzie C. Cervenka. "Dietary Therapy Is the Best Option for Refractory Nonsurgical

Epilepsy." Epilepsia, vol. 56, no. 9, 2015, pp. 1325–1329., doi: 10.1111/epi.13075.

16. Ferriss, Timothy. "Podcast – The Tim Ferriss Show #117: Dom D'Agostino, Ph.D. on Fasting, Ketosis, and The End of Cancer." The Blog of Author Tim Ferriss, 3 Nov. 2015, tim.blog/podcast/.

17. Feyter, Henk M. De, et al. "A Ketogenic Diet Increases Transport and Oxidation of Ketone Bodies in RG2 and 9L Gliomas without Affecting Tumor Growth." Neuro-Oncology, vol. 18, no. 8, Mar. 2016, pp. 1079–1087., doi:10.1093/neuonc/now088.

18. Fine, Eugene J, et al. "Acetoacetate Reduces Growth and ATP Concentration in Cancer Cell Lines Which over-Express Uncoupling Protein 2." Cancer Cell International, vol. 9, no. 1, 2009, p. 14., doi: 10.1186/1475-2867-9-14.

19. Fine, Eugene J., et al. "Carbohydrate Restriction in Patients with Advanced Cancer: a Protocol to Assess Safety and Feasibility with an Accompanying Hypothesis." Community Oncology, vol. 5, no. 1, 2008, pp. 22–26., doi:10.1016/s1548-5315(11)70179-6.

20. Fine, Eugene J., et al. "Targeting Insulin Inhibition as a Metabolic Therapy in Advanced Cancer: A Pilot Safety and Feasibility Dietary Trial in 10 Patients." Nutrition, vol. 28, no. 10, 2012, pp. 1028–1035., doi:10.1016/j.nut.2012.05.001.

21. Fogelholm, Mikael. "Faculty of 1000 Evaluation for Meta-Analysis of Prospective Cohort Studies Evaluating the Association of Saturated Fat with Cardiovascular Disease." F1000 - Post-Publication Peer Review of the Biomedical Literature, Nov. 2010, doi:10.3410/f. 1947957.1501056.

22. Forsythe, Cassandra E., et al. "Comparison of Low Fat and Low Carbohydrate Diets on Circulating Fatty Acid Composition and

Markers of Inflammation." Lipids, vol. 43, no. 1, 2007, pp. 65–77., doi:10.1007/s11745-007-3132-7.

23. Forsythe, Cassandra E., et al. "Limited Effect of Dietary Saturated Fat on Plasma Saturated Fat in the Context of a Low Carbohydrate Diet." Lipids, vol. 45, no. 10, July 2010, pp. 947–962., doi: 10.1007/s11745-010-3467-3.

24. Franklin, Carl, and Richard Morris. "Ketogenic Forums." Ketogenic Forums, www.ketogenicforums.com/.

25. Fung, Jason. "Blog." Intensive Dietary Management (IDM), idmprogram.com/blog/.

26. Fung, Jason. The Obesity Code: Unlocking the Secrets of Weight Loss. Greystone Books, 2016.

27. Goldberg, Emily L., et al. "Beta-Hydroxybutyrate Deactivates Neutrophil NLRP3 Inflammasome to Relieve Gout Flares." Cell Reports, vol. 18, no. 9, 2017, pp. 2077–2087., doi:10.1016/j.celrep. 2017.02.004.

28. Hertz, Leif, et al. "Effects of Ketone Bodies in Alzheimer's Disease in Relation to Neural Hypometabolism, Beta-Amyloid Toxicity, and Astrocyte Function." Journal of Neurochemistry, vol. 134, no. 1, 2015, pp. 7–20., doi:10.1111/jnc.13107.

29. Jeffery, Mark. "MD Anderson Cancer Center." The Lancet Oncology, vol. 2, no. 3, 2001, p. 186., doi:10.1016/ s1470-2045(00)00270-9.

30. Just, Tino, et al. "Cephalic Phase Insulin Release in Healthy Humans after Taste Stimulation?" Appetite, vol. 51, no. 3, 2008, pp. 622–627., doi:10.1016/j.appet.2008.04.271.

31. Kawamura, Masahito. "Ketogenic Diet in a Hippocampal Slice." Oxford Medicine Online, 2016, doi:10.1093/med/ 9780190497996.003.0021.

32. Kelley, Sarah Aminoff, and Eric Heath Kossoff. "How Effective Is the Ketogenic Diet for Electrical Status Epilepticus of Sleep?" Epilepsy Research, vol. 127, 2016, pp. 339–343., doi:10.1016/j.eplepsyres.2016.09.018.

33. Kerndt, Peter R., et al. "Fasting: The History, Pathophysiology and Complications." THE WESTERN JOURNAL OF MEDICINE, vol. 137, no. 5, Nov. 1982, pp. 379–399.

34. Keys, Ancel, and Margaret Keys. How to Eat Well and Stay Well. Doubleday, 1959.

35. Kindwall, Eric P., and Harry T. Whelan. Hyperbaric Medicine Practice. Best Pub. Co., 2008.

36. Klement, Rainer J., and Reinhart A. Sweeney. "Impact of a Ketogenic Diet Intervention during Radiotherapy on Body Composition: I. Initial Clinical Experience with Six Prospectively Studied Patients." BMC Research Notes, vol. 9, no. 1, May 2016, doi:10.1186/s13104-016-1959-9.

37. Klement, Rainer J., et al. "Anti-Tumor Effects of Ketogenic Diets in Mice: A Meta-Analysis." Plos One, vol. 11, no. 5, Sept. 2016, doi:10.1371/journal.pone.0155050.

38. Kossoff, Eric. Ketogenic Diets: Treatments for Epilepsy and Other Disorders. Readhowyouwant.com Ltd, 2012.

39. Kratz, Mario, et al. "The Relationship between High-Fat Dairy Consumption and Obesity, Cardiovascular, and Metabolic Disease." European Journal of Nutrition, vol. 52, no. 1, 2012, pp. 1–24., doi:10.1007/s00394-012-0418-1.

40. Li, Donghui. "Molecular Epidemiology." M. D. Anderson Solid Tumor Oncology Series Pancreatic Cancer, pp. 3–13., doi: 10.1007/0-387-21600-6_1.

41. Longo, Valter. LONGEVITY DIET. PENGUIN BOOKS, 2018.

42. Lorenzo, C. Di, et al. "Migraine Improvement during Short Lasting Ketogenesis: a Proof-of-Concept Study." European Journal of Neurology, vol. 22, no. 1, 2014, pp. 170–177., doi:10.1111/ene.12550.

43. Lowe, Aileen, et al. "Neurogenesis and Precursor Cell Differences in the Dorsal and Ventral Adult Canine Hippocampus." Neuroscience Letters, vol. 593, 2015, pp. 107–113., doi:10.1016/j.neulet. 2015.03.017.

44. Lussier, Danielle M., et al. "Enhanced Immunity in a Mouse Model of Malignant Glioma Is Mediated by a Therapeutic Ketogenic Diet." BMC Cancer, vol. 16, no. 1, 2016, doi:10.1186/ s12885-016-2337-7.

45. Maalouf, M, et al. "The Neuroprotective Properties of Calorie Restriction, the Ketogenic Diet, and Ketone Bodies." Brain Research Reviews., U.S. National Library of Medicine, Mar. 2009, www.ncbi.nlm.nih.gov/pubmed/18845187.

46. Masino, Susan A., and David N. Ruskin. "Ketogenic Diets and Pain." Journal of Child Neurology, vol. 28, no. 8, 2013, pp. 993–1001., doi:10.1177/0883073813487595.

47. Masino, Susan A., et al. "A Ketogenic Diet Suppresses Seizures in Mice through Adenosine A1 Receptors." Journal of Clinical Investigation, vol. 121, no. 7, Jan. 2011, pp. 2679–2683., doi: 10.1172/jci57813.

48. Mavropoulos, J. C., et al. "The Effects of Varying Dietary Carbohydrate and Fat Content on Survival in a Murine LNCaP Prostate Cancer Xenograft Model." Cancer Prevention Research, vol. 2, no. 6, 2009, pp. 557–565., doi:10.1158/1940-6207.capr-08-0188.

49. Mente, Andrew, et al. "A Systematic Review of the Evidence Supporting a Causal Link Between Dietary Factors and Coronary

Heart Disease." Archives of Internal Medicine, vol. 169, no. 7, 2009, p. 659., doi:10.1001/archinternmed.2009.38.

50. Nabbout, Rima. "FIRES and IHHE: Delineation of the Syndromes." Epilepsia, vol. 54, 2013, pp. 54–56., doi:10.1111/epi.12278.

51. Ness, A. "Diet, Nutrition and the Prevention of Chronic Diseases. WHO Technical Report Series 916. Report of a Joint WHO/FSA Expert Consultation." International Journal of Epidemiology, vol. 33, no. 4, 2004, pp. 914–915., doi:10.1093/ije/dyh209.

52. Nestle, M. "Mediterranean Diets: Historical and Research Overview." The American Journal of Clinical Nutrition, vol. 61, no. 6, Jan. 1995, doi:10.1093/ajcn/61.6.1313s.

53. Newport, Mary T. Alzheimer's Disease: What If There Was a Cure? the Story of Ketones. Basic Health, 2013.

54. "Nobel Prize Honors Autophagy Discovery." Cancer Discovery, vol. 6, no. 12, 2016, pp. 1298–1299., doi:10.1158/2159-8290.cd-nb2016-127.

55. Nuttall, F. Q., and M. C. Gannon. "Plasma Glucose and Insulin Response to Macronutrients in Nondiabetic and NIDDM Subjects." Diabetes Care, vol. 14, no. 9, Jan. 1991, pp. 824–838., doi: 10.2337/diacare.14.9.824.

56. Ogawa, Chikako, et al. "Autopsy Findings of a Patient with Acute Encephalitis and Refractory, Repetitive Partial Seizures." Seizure, vol. 35, 2016, pp. 80–82., doi:10.1016/j.seizure.2016.01.005.

57. Palmer, Joshua D., et al. "Brain Tumours." Re-Irradiation: New Frontiers Medical Radiology, 2016, pp. 127–142., doi: 10.1007/174_2016_66.

58. Reeves, Sue, et al. "Experimental Manipulation of Breakfast in Normal and Overweight/Obese Participants Is Associated with

Changes to Nutrient and Energy Intake Consumption Patterns." Physiology & Behavior, vol. 133, 2014, pp. 130–135., doi:10.1016/j.physbeh.2014.05.015.

59. Seyfried, Thomas N. Cancer as a Metabolic Disease: on the Origin, Management, and Prevention of Cancer. Wiley-Blackwell, 2012.

60. Seyfried, Thomas N., et al. "Is the Restricted Ketogenic Diet a Viable Alternative to the Standard of Care for Managing Malignant Brain Cancer?" Epilepsy Research, vol. 100, no. 3, 2012, pp. 310–326., doi:10.1016/j.eplepsyres.2011.06.017.

61. Seyfried, Thomas N., et al. "Metabolic Therapy: A New Paradigm for Managing Malignant Brain Cancer." Cancer Letters, vol. 356, no. 2, 2015, pp. 289–300., doi:10.1016/j.canlet.2014.07.015.

62. Sherwood, Louis M., et al. "Starvation in Man." New England Journal of Medicine, vol. 282, no. 12, 1970, pp. 668–675., doi: 10.1056/nejm197003192821209.

63. Shine, N., and D. Say. "Effectiveness of Ketone Level on Seizure Control." Journal of the American Dietetic Association, vol. 97, no. 9, 1997, doi:10.1016/s0002-8223(97)00497-5.

64. Silva-Nichols, Helena B., et al. "Atps-77 The Ketone Body Beta-Hydroxybutyrate Radiosensitizes Glioblastoma Multiforme Stem Cells." Neuro-Oncology, vol. 17, no. suppl 5, 2015, doi:10.1093/neuonc/nov204.77.

65. Simeone, Timothy A., et al. "Ketone Bodies as Anti-Seizure Agents." Neurochemical Research, vol. 42, no. 7, Oct. 2017, pp. 2011–2018., doi:10.1007/s11064-017-2253-5.

66. Siri-Tarino, P. W, et al. "Meta-Analysis of Prospective Cohort Studies Evaluating the Association of Saturated Fat with Cardiovascular Disease." American Journal of Clinical Nutrition, vol. 91, no. 3, 2010, pp. 535–546., doi:10.3945/ajcn.2009.27725.

67. Smyl, Christopher. "Ketogenic Diet and Cancer - a Perspective." Metabolism in Cancer Recent Results in Cancer Research, 2016, pp. 233–240., doi:10.1007/978-3-319-42118-6_11.

68. Stubbs, James, et al. "Macronutrients, Feeding Behavior, and Weight Control in Humans." Appetite and Food Intake, 2008, pp. 295–322., doi:10.1201/9781420047844.ch16.

69. Tiukinhoy, Susan, and Carolyn L. Rochester. "Low-Fat Dietary Pattern And Risk Of Cardiovascular Disease-The Women's Health Initiative Randomized Controlled Dietary Modification Trial." Journal of Cardiopulmonary Rehabilitation, vol. 26, no. 3, 2006, pp. 191–192., doi:10.1097/00008483-200605000-00015.

70. Toth, Csaba, and Maria Schimmer, Zsófia Clemens. "Complete Cessation of Recurrent Cervical Intraepithelial Neoplasia (CIN) by the Paleolithic Ketogenic Diet: A Case Report." Journal of Cancer Research and Treatment, vol. 6, no. 1, Apr. 2018, pp. 1–5., doi: 10.12691/jcrt-6-1-1.

71. Toth, Csaba, and Zsófia Clemens. "Halted Progression of Soft Palate Cancer in a Patient Treated with the Paleolithic Ketogenic Diet Alone: A 20-Months Follow-Up." American Journal of Medical Case Reports, vol. 4, no. 8, 2016, pp. 288–292.

72. Vergati, Matteo, et al. "Ketogenic Diet and Other Dietary Intervention Strategies in the Treatment of Cancer." Current Medicinal Chemistry, vol. 24, no. 12, 2017, doi: 10.2174/0929867324666170116122915.

73. Volek, Jeff, and Stephen D. Phinney. The Art and Science of Low Carbohydrate Living: an Expert Guide to Making the Life-Saving Benefits of Carbohydrate Restriction Sustainable and Enjoyable. Beyond Obesity, 2011.

74. Volek, Jeff S., et al. "Effects of Dietary Carbohydrate Restriction versus Low-Fat Diet on Flow-Mediated Dilation." Metabolism,

vol. 58, no. 12, 2009, pp. 1769–1777., doi:10.1016/j.metabol. 2009.06.005.

75. Volek, Jeff S, et al. "Low-Carbohydrate Diets Promote a More Favorable Body Composition Than Low-Fat Diets." Strength and Conditioning Journal, vol. 32, no. 1, 2010, pp. 42–47., doi:10.1519/ ssc.0b013e3181c16c41.

76. Westman, Eric C. ADAPT Program: a Low Carbohydrate, Ketogenic Diet Manual. Adapt Your Life, Inc., 2015.

77. Wheless, James W. "History and Origin of the Ketogenic Diet." Epilepsy and the Ketogenic Diet, 2004, pp. 31–50., doi: 10.1007/978-1-59259-808-3_2.

78. Winter, Sebastian F., et al. "Role of Ketogenic Metabolic Therapy in Malignant Glioma: A Systematic Review." Critical Reviews in Oncology/Hematology, vol. 112, 2017, pp. 41–58., doi: 10.1016/j.critrevonc.2017.02.016.

79. Woolf, Eric C., and Adrienne C. Scheck. "The Ketogenic Diet for the Adjuvant Treatment of Malignant Brain Tumors." Bioactive Nutraceuticals and Dietary Supplements in Neurological and Brain Disease, 2015, pp. 125–135., doi:10.1016/b978-0-12-411462-3.00013-8.

80. Wyatt, Holly R., et al. "Long-Term Weight Loss and Breakfast in Subjects in the National Weight Control Registry." Obesity Research, vol. 10, no. 2, 2002, pp. 78–82., doi:10.1038/oby.2002.13.

81. Zinn, Caryn, et al. "Ketogenic Diet Benefits Body Composition and Well-Being but Not Performance in a Pilot Case Study of New Zealand Endurance Athletes." Journal of the International Society of Sports Nutrition, BioMed Central, 12 July 2017, jissn.biomedcentral.com/articles/10.1186/s12970-017-0180-0.

www.BozMD.com

Make smart choices, Not sacrifices.

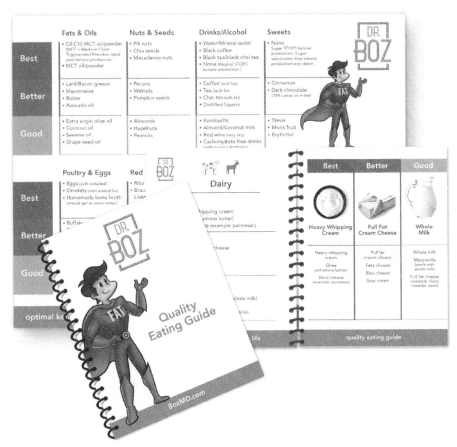

To enter ketosis, you need to know which foods and beverages will spark your body's natural energy production. This Pocket Guide & Fridge Chart will step you through foods that are good Better and BEST for your keto journey. At the grocery story or dining out, this reference will help you make better choices one decision at a time.

QUALITY EATING POCKET GUIDE & FRIDGE CHART

<u>Quality Eating Guide</u>: [Size:4 x 5.5 inch] Take this handy pocket guide with you on every trip to the market or restaurant. There are 30 pages of Good, Better, and Best food options. Let me walk you through the gradual improvement of your food choices. This guide is printed on water resistant, non-tearable, synthetic paper for maximum durability. Change happens one decision at a time. Use this guide to move to the next best decision.

<u>Fridge Magnet</u>: [Size:11 x 8.5 inch] Feature this laminated eating guide on your refrigerator – or any magnetic service – as an easy-to-use reminder of your successful keto-journey. My favorite reviews of this tool have come from those who hung this in the kitchen area at work. Watch the discussions begin!

Special Thanks to:

Mark & Dawn Aspaas
Adriana Avelle
Peggy Craig
Pete Hansen
Jade Hendricks
Terry Kjergaard
Bettie and John Mathis
Ryan Myer
Patrick & Jennifer Rosenstiel
Becky Scheideler
Lauren Stranahan
Doug Tschetter
Luke Tunge
Kerri Tunge

... and the thousands of patients that have
blessed my life by inviting me into theirs.

Made in the USA
Monee, IL
08 July 2020